Powerful Occupational Therapists

Powerful Occupational Therapists examines the life and times of a small group of occupational therapy leaders and scholars in a post-1950s America, to market their profession as one of increasing importance. Participating in the 1950s rehabilitation, the 1960s equal rights, and the 1970s women's movements, these innovators, being primarily women, aimed to define themselves as having professional and scientific authority that was distinct from the male-dominated medical model. The community of therapists faced challenges such as that of retaining the appearance of being "ladylike" whilst doing "unladylike" tasks. This book describes the personal experiences of 12 differing occupational therapists and it identifies how a group of them strengthened and developed the profession in the face of diverse challenges. This volume would be of interest to those studying occupational therapy, women and medicine and the history of medicine.

This book was originally published as a special issue of *Occupational Therapy in Mental Health*.

Christine Olga Peters is recognized for advancing occupational therapy history. She has presented occupational therapy history internationally and at the United Nations. She received the American Occupational Therapy Association (AOTA) and American Occupational Therapy Foundation (AOTF) Leadership Fellowship and the AOTF Certificate of Appreciation. She is also a Fellow of American Occupational Therapy Association (AOTA).

Powerful Occupational Therapists

A Community of Professionals, 1950–1980

Christine Olga Peters

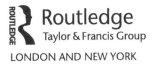
Routledge
Taylor & Francis Group

LONDON AND NEW YORK

First published 2013
by Routledge
2 Park Square, Milton Park, Abingdon, Oxon, OX14 4RN

Simultaneously published in the USA and Canada
by Routledge
711 Third Avenue, New York, NY 10017

First issued in paperback 2017

Routledge is an imprint of the Taylor & Francis Group, an informa business

This book is a reproduction of *Occupational Therapy in Mental Health*, vol. 27, issue 3-4. The Publisher requests to those authors who may be citing this book to state, also, the bibliographical details of the special issue on which the book was based.

British Library Cataloguing in Publication Data
A catalogue record for this book is available from the British Library

Typeset in Garamond
By Taylor & Francis Books

Publisher's Note
The publisher would like to make readers aware that the chapters in this book may be referred to as articles as they are identical to the articles published in the special issue. The publisher accepts responsibility for any inconsistencies that may have arisen in the course of preparing this volume for print.

ISBN 13: 978-1-138-10864-6 (pbk)
ISBN 13: 978-0-415-63185-3 (hbk)

Contents

Citation Information

The chapters in this book were originally published in *Occupational Therapy in Mental Health*, volume 27, issue 3-4 (November 2011). When citing this material, please use the original page numbering for each article, as follows:

Foreword
Occupational Therapy in Mental Health, volume 27, issue 3-4 (November 2011) pp. 197-198

Section 1
Changing in Response to Science
Occupational Therapy in Mental Health, volume 27, issue 3-4 (November 2011) pp. 199-218

Section 2
The Study
Occupational Therapy in Mental Health, volume 27, issue 3-4 (November 2011) pp. 218-231

Section 3
Community of Therapists
Occupational Therapy in Mental Health, volume 27, issue 3-4 (November 2011) pp. 231-245

Section 4
Community Groupings and Portraits
Occupational Therapy in Mental Health, volume 27, issue 3-4 (November 2011) pp. 245-280

Section 5
Political Movers and Sustainers
Occupational Therapy in Mental Health, volume 27, issue 3-4 (November 2011) pp. 280-327

Section 6
The Dilemma of Philosophy and Science
Occupational Therapy in Mental Health, volume 27, issue 3-4 (November 2011) pp. 327-355

Section 7

Professionalizing: Occupational Therapy and Social Movements
Occupational Therapy in Mental Health, volume 27, issue 3-4 (November 2011) pp. 355-381

Section 8

Occupational Therapy's Past Influences Its Present, and Conclusion
Occupational Therapy in Mental Health, volume 27, issue 3-4 (November 2011) pp. 381-385

Foreword

Since my initial writing of *Powerful Occupational Therapists: A Community of Professionals, 1950–1980*, certain individuals you will read about have died. All advanced in years, their having given their words and personal documents to this researcher makes their contributions more cherished. For example, Dr. Robert K. Bing dealt with hospitalizations during the study, and when able, was back to participating fully. His contribution to this work was an example of his commitment to the preservation of occupational therapy history, literally to the end of his life. Another, Gail S. Fidler, gave her last oral history as part of this study, and although weathered with health concerns, she was enlivened during our days together, with her all too familiar tilt of the head backwards when she laughed, particularly when she challenged the state of occupational therapy.

Because of more recent losses, I have chosen to acknowledge these individuals in a foreword, and dedicate the work not only to them, but to the community of occupational therapists who moved a profession forward at an often overlooked time in the profession's history: 1950 until 1980. These therapists who have died are alphabetically listed; Robert K. Bing (deceased in 2003), Marion Crampton (deceased 2011), Gail S. Fidler (deceased in 2005), Ann P. Grady (deceased in 2012), Mary Reilly (deceased in 2012), Carlotta Welles (deceased in 2010), and Ruth Brunyate Wiemer (deceased in 2009). Two spouses are worthy of remembrance: Dr. Joseph "Joe" Paul Llorens (deceased in 2006), who, although ill during the oral history visit, remained vibrantly alive in the many paintings that he painted that graced the Llorens living room walls. I remember our quiet chats in his favorite room outfitted with a television and comfortable chairs, while we reminisced about the early 1980s, when I was his wife Lela Lloren's student. I would also like to acknowledge the passing of Eugene (Gene) Gilfoyle (deceased 2010), who was the husband of occupational therapist Elnora Gilfoyle. A strong advocate for the profession, Gene also participated in sharing stories of his memories of his wife's peer group that brought these pages to life.

Other recent changes included Martha Kirkland and Nedra Gillette's retirement from the American Occupational Therapy Foundation. Ms. Kirkland, in her leadership of the American Occupational Therapy Foundation, now has a Leadership Award named in her honor from the foundation. Ms. Gillette, since the study, became a recipient of the American Occupational Therapy's Award of Merit.

Their stories are a representative sample of powerful pioneers and players in an occupational therapy arena. Growing from this work, I have had the opportunity to engage in a study with Dr Evelyn Andersson funded by Midwestern University about Ms. Lorna Jean King, a contemporary of Drs. A. Jean Ayres and Margaret Rood. As the circle expands, adding more to the community of occupational therapy pioneers from the 1950s through 1980, it is clear that the complexities of historical richness darken like a fine patina.

Christine Olga Peters, PhD, OTR/L, FAOTA Consultant
Sound Beach, New York

A powerful community of therapists changed occupational therapy in the United States between 1950 until 1980. These innovators, primarily women, strategically positioned themselves to market the emerging profession. These therapists, categorized as theorists and futurists, political movers and new and old guard sustainers, determined occupational therapy's direction. Participating in the 1950s rehabilitation, the 1960s equal rights, and the 1970s women's movements, the community of therapists separated from the male-dominated medical model to gain professional and scientific authority. An internal tension arouse between those therapists embracing an objective, and arguably male, science and those supporting a characteristically feminine caring philosophical base.

SECTION I: CHANGING IN RESPONSE TO SCIENCE

Theory developers and tradition breakers describe a small group of occupational therapists as guiding a relatively new, and often overlooked rehabilitation health profession, as occupational therapy became a science-based profession between 1950 and 1980 in the United States. Three research questions guided my inquiry about occupational therapy's road to science.

1. How did occupational therapy's supporting body of knowledge affect the development of the profession between 1950 and 1980?

2. Who were the occupational therapy scholars and leaders, and why did they support professionalism?
3. What occupational therapists' beliefs and actions shaped occupational therapy's evolution as a science-based profession?

Occupational therapy's evolution in the larger story about the history of professions, particularly female-dominated professions, provides an understanding of how professions develop a theoretical rationale for practice. In that process, they professionalize. Curiously, a dilemma develops when a female profession embraces something considered to be as decidedly male as science. This process was not easily executed in occupational therapy. Occupationaltherapy attempted to feminize its science both by using scholarly merit and female strategies like community-building. This proved a viable strategy for women working in "semi-professional" (Etzioni, 1969) health professions like occupational therapy and nursing, who were caught in a conflict between their traditional nurturing caregiver stereotype and the desire for career mobility perhaps modeled after men.[1]

Occupational therapy's embrace of science, and the thesis of this work, came not from the importance of a knowledge base as a key to professionalization, but from the commitment and power of a group of therapists who positioned themselves in strategic arenas to market the emerging profession. I argue that scholarship and a debate about a scientific basis for practice alone were not enough for occupational therapy to gain professional authority. Rather, well-placed, academically talented, or politically astute women knew that legitimizing the profession meant professional viability. Reflecting the 1950s in her oral history, occupational therapist Gail Fidler stated "Well, it was scarcely well-known, so as an OT, you were a minority, no matter how it played out. Because no one, very few, other than OTs themselves knew about OT." (Fidler/Peters oral history, March 6–7, 2003, lines 37–40)

Like an unread book on a shelf, knowledge for knowledge's sake was a longer-range goal and not pragmatic enough for a post-1950s occupational therapy. Playing out in various venues, strategic placement meant partnerships, membership or competition with medicine, similar healthcare professions, political and policy-making organizations, education, and the military. Occupational therapists entered these relationships overtly or covertly, as a core group or individually, sometimes either accepted or ostracized by occupational therapy's leadership. These therapists making steps to a larger professional world were the real leaders and scholars driving the profession.

During that time period, 1950 to 1980, occupational therapy needed visibility for viability. Occupational therapy held too small a place in a competitive health care market to thrive. Viability as understood by the larger membership related to more practical needs characterized as a "manpower shortage," or patient load, rather than to the building of theoretical foundations. Then why did occupational therapy's intellectuals and leading practitioners prioritize developing and contributing to a scientific body of knowledge? Secondly, was this emerging knowledge base scientific or philosophical in nature? This historical dilemma continues today. Today's scholars continue to discuss the pros and cons of basic versus applied occupational therapy research and practice, echoing threads from the past (AOTF, 2000a; Clark et al., 1993; Mosey, 1993; Parham, 1998).

A select group of occupational therapy's community of therapists took an atypical path toward creating knowledge, when 1950s women typically did not work outside of the home. These therapists became scientists, scholars, leaders, and administrators; roles usually reserved for men at the time. This community had insiders and outsiders, or therapists accepted within an inner circle and others externalized, by their choice or by exclusion. Standing and placement in the community remained unstated but known. Shrewd leaders taking the insider track knew the importance of people, places, and opportunities while promoting their beliefs that occupational therapy uniquely helped society. Occupational therapy's leaders, master practitioners, and managers navigated a predominantly female profession that today remains 94% women (AOTA, 2001a, 2001b). Mentoring mostly women and some men brought gender issues and feminizing leadership styles (Bennis, 1989; Burke & De Poy, 1991; Kirkpatrick & Locke, 1991; Roberston, 1992; Rogers, 1982; Rozier, 1994; Schemm & Bross, 1995).

The outsider theorists used the published word as their occupational therapy building tool rather than their political placement. The outsiders were loners by choice or were ostracized by other community members. Taken as a whole, these peer-identified brilliant scholars helped occupational therapy create a body of theoretical knowledge. Beyond knowledge development, they shaped the profession. Their stories illuminated how change occurred, and if left untold, could have been lost.

Historical occupational therapy analysis relating to the professional evolution of knowledge and scholarship in a predominantly female profession is sparse, particularly in the years between 1950 and 1980. Schwartz (1992a), an occupational therapy historian, views occupational therapy's historical body of knowledge as emerging. I argue that few scholars have tackled occupational therapy historical analysis and synthesis at the level of complexity needed to understand how answering questions from the past can contribute to formulating questions today.

While there has been some interest in capturing occupational therapy history as seen in the American Occupational Therapy Association's (AOTA's) and the American Occupational Therapy Foundation's (AOTF's) joint effort to complete a written history project in the 1980s, that effort was budgeted at $21, 575, a conservative amount compared to that needed. Efforts after that time stalled or lacked continued funding (Kirkland, August 13, 1987 memorandum to AOTA Executive Board regarding: Plan for completing the written history of occupational therapy, Bing, private papers; Schwartz & Colman, 1988).

Developing a realistic scope for the work, Martha Kirkland, the Executive Director of AOTF, consulted historian Susan Reverby, PhD, Director of Women's Studies, Wellesley College.[2] Kirkland, writing to AOTA President and occupational therapy historian Robert K. Bing, characterized the written history project, as the impossible dream, stating:

> I am writing to bring you up-to-date on our progress toward the Written History of Occupational Therapy, also known as the 'impossible dream.' This has been a star-crossed project, having been off to several false starts. I understand that you have proposed a (Eleanor Clarke Slagle) play idea to the (AOTA) National Conference Committee. I think Willie (Wilma West) was also smitten with the creative idea because she appeared in the 1955 or so version. (Kirkland to Bing, August 25, 1987, Bing private papers)

Kirkland was accurate in her assessment about how difficult it was to compile occupational therapy's history, a long standing concern. For example, occupational therapy leader Myra McDaniel accepted the AOTA's Council on Development's charge (Resolution 210) in 1968 to study the Association's development. McDaniel organized ten years of records and proposed a 15-chapter volume covering the history of the profession and the association. This evolved into the written history project that went through numerous false starts. McDaniel's 1960s study changed in 1976 when the allocated funds were funneled to AOTA's Resolution 488-76 to produce AOTA historical materials on videotape. The AOTA Executive Board then designated that $60,000, over a three-year period, be used to reactivate the written history project. This did not occur. Rather, in May 1978, Resolution 526-78 was passed to form an archives committee. The archives committee chaired by Robert K. Bing completed the task of cataloging occupational therapy historical records until 1978 (Bowman & Scherer, n.d.). The AOTA Executive Board, in August, 1978, passed a motion to form a written history committee that was co-chaired by therapists Helen Hopkins, Ruth Griffin, and Betty Cox. Under this committee's charge, a written history symposium occurred at AOTA's Annual Conferences, in Portland, Oregon (April 14–15, 1983), and Kansas City, Missouri, (May 4–5, 1984), where occupational thera-pists presented their monograph series of unpublished papers. I believe this was likely too small a venue for a potentially key project. This summary illus-trates the thwarted efforts that occurred on an organizational level between 1968 and 1987, and the need for documenting and capturing occupational therapy's past. Secondly, what other professional priorities took precedence over funding occupational therapy history projects?

There is also limited information about how occupational therap-ists became scholars and leaders, particularly from a historical stance that specifically examines who these people were, why they became scholars and leaders, and how their gender, class, and race influenced their careers and work. Although there is a small repository of oral histories of occupational therapy scholars and leaders located in the profession's national archive, questions about how these people contributed to occupational therapy's science-base were not asked. Obtaining this information directly from those occupational therapists who made significant contributions through oral histories has broadened our understanding of this period.

Finally, this study was needed for two reasons: one grounded in occupational therapy present, another to recapture the past. History allows us to study and gain insight about why and how decisions were made in a profession's past (Rampolla, 2001; Stattel, 1977). Occupational therapists Schwartz and Colman (1988) state that a student of occupational therapy history must "unwind inconsistencies of the past" (p. 244) to develop coherent pictures. In this study I draw on numerous pictures from the past to bring to life this time in occupational therapy history through existing documents and personal stories. More vividly, readers are introduced to the people who lived and made occupational therapy, helping it evolve into today's profession.

Understanding post-1950s occupational therapy is about understanding the therapists who practiced and promoted the profession at a time when the public knew health care as physicians, nurses, and social workers. Ten occupational therapists responsible for changing occupational therapy shared their public and private career accounts. Unprecedented, and also remarkable in their telling of the stories, these therapists represent occupational therapy's core movers and shakers, each having 50-year legacies and commitment to one profession. Unanimously, these women and men coming from contrasting backgrounds and geographic locations shared a mutual goal: to professionalize occupational therapy.

What was so seductive about occupational therapy to those who practiced it? On the surface, occupational therapists—largely characterized as crafts ladies or basket-weavers keeping patients busy—practiced simplistic work having minimal theoretical rationale. Secondarily characterized, occupational therapists kept patients engaged doing handcrafts while others, such as doctors, performed the real work of medicine. Not well-understood, patients who received occupational therapy improved (Meyer, 1922). Occupational therapists knew their functional work was more than diversional or busy activity. Whatever occupational therapists did, although not clearly understood by many, it worked. This enigmatic profession attracted talented women and men, some ready to take on the needed work to educate not only patients, but also the larger health care system, thus giving rise to a growing profession.

Informally forming a community of therapists, they dedicated their professional and private time to building lifelong relationships within the community while professionalizing occupational therapy. Fueled by countless volunteer hours in addition to their employed hours away from family and private life, using their personal money when needed, this nucleus of therapists helped build a profession. Some therapists captured federal grants or military stipends that funded their master's and doctoral education, spurring occupational therapy research. Other federal and state funding sources supported experimental clinical programs and workshops. Findings from these projects were often published, adding to occupational therapy literature.

Therapists' roads varied. Some, at times, forfeited their career security by speaking out in disagreement. Others worked effectively along established lines. Some worked with other occupational therapists in large hospital settings. Others worked as the only occupational therapist in various multidisciplinary teams. Others worked in federal and state agencies as educators and clinical or academic administrators, or sole practitioners. Whatever their career path, they demonstrated occupational therapy's value to others, sharing their beliefs.

How was this community different from the 1917 occupational therapy leaders and founders that I will be discussing in the next section? White male physicians and administrators, barring one exception, Eleanor Clarke Slagle, mentored and managed occupational therapy's first 30 years. These men held high positions in the national occupational therapy organization, published occupational therapy journals and books, and supervised practice. Breaking from tradition, occupational therapy theorist's created their own, rather than physicians', rationale for treatment. This new intellectual autonomy proved freeing for some scholars, evident in their authoring books, rather than physician authored texts. Others entered physician-therapist partnerships, particularly in the 1950s and 1960s, seeing medicine as a foundation to occupational therapy's science base. An understandable move considering partnerships helped anchor the developing occupational therapy profession. Who really was interested in occupational therapy's knowledge other than the therapists themselves, or the physicians who saw themselves as founding fathers who initially developed that knowledge? Ultimately, the road to science was more an interest of a few compared with the many, namely the community of therapists, some of whom you will meet in these pages. The primarily female 1950s–1980 community of therapists formed networks that they described as family or a sisterhood, giving rise to a powerful feminism.

Occupational Therapy's Beginnings

Occupational therapy's back road to science draws from early 20th century American ideology touting a puritan work value and healthy habits. Philosophically, therapists viewed meaningful work or occupation as important for a productive life. How therapists achieved these ideals or a more scientific approach to occupation was happenstance at first, or trial and error. Using arts and crafts kept patients' hands and minds active, ultimately forming healthy habits and balance in life (Licht, 1950; Meyer, 1922).

The idea that human occupation counteracts illness and character flaws was traced to ancient Greek and Roman philosophers. Socrates argued that "all human activities depend on the soul, and those of the soul itself depend on wisdom to be good" (Plato, 1976, p. 22). Plato's student Aristotle continued this thinking, stating, "every art and inquiry, and similarly every action and pursuit is thought to aim at some good," (Aristotle, 1925/1980, p. 1). Modern history roots links occupational therapy principles to 18th century Europe and the once shackled mentally ill. Unchaining these patients, French psychiatrist Philippe Pinel prescribed exercise and manual occupation. Similarly, Quaker and mental health advocate Tuke also promoted work treatment for the mentally ill in England (Bing, 1981).

By mid-19th century the moral treatment movement had taken hold in the United States with new work therapy programs established at McLean Asylum in Boston and the Bloomingdale Asylum for the Insane in New York. Pioneer American psychiatrist Benjamin Rush identified a need for craft teachers, supporting diversional occupation for practical rather than scientific reasons (AOTA, 1967). Filling a need, training schools such as the Chicago School of Civics and Philanthropy headed by Julia Lathrop in 1906, offered courses emphasizing handicrafts, exercise, and play. These courses were designed for mental health nursing supervisors, attendants, and social workers. One student, Eleanor Clarke Slagle, Director of the Chicago School in 1915, came from a politically connected New York family. Slagle, a mental health activist, administrator, and social worker, began meeting and working with like-minded people who supported occupational patient activities (Dunton, 1947).

Prior to World War I, and consistent with the arts and crafts movement in this country, therapeutic crafts training courses grew. Psychiatrist and skilled craftsman William Rush Dunton, Jr., a cousin to Benjamin Rush, taught one such course in 1911 at the Sheppard and Enoch Pratt Hospital in Baltimore. Dunton used metal, reed work, and printing press activities when working with patients. Susan Tracy, another crafts advocate, discovered when she was a nursing student at Columbia University in New York that patients recovered more quickly when they were occupied. Formalizing her thoughts, Tracy published in 1910 "Studies on Invalid Occupation," a crafts training manual for nurses. Presenting an idea which proved to be controversial years later, Tracy believed that occupational therapists should be nurses (Quiroga, 1995).

George Barton, an architect and self-made therapist seeking his own health, established Consolation House, in Clifton Springs, New York at a time parallel to Dunton's and Tracy's work. Clifton Springs flourished as a healing summer community, nestled between Susan B. Anthony's homestead in Rochester, the suffragist's stomping grounds in Seneca Falls, and the Roycraft Arts and Crafts community in East Aurora, founded in 1895 by writer and philosopher Elbert Hubbard. Early 20th century upstate New York's progressive landscape merged medicine, the women's movement, and the arts and crafts movement, and provided a backdrop for occupational therapy's founding.

Barton, buying a two-story, white pillar, wood-frame home, created a workshop where patients could learn profitable occupations. Barton, who expanded the arts and crafts movement to patient care, is credited for creating the term occupational therapy (Quiroga, 1995). Consolation House had a full workshop behind the main house, where crafts construction varied from furniture building to weaving. Occupational therapy flourished at Consolation House and the nearby Clifton Springs Sanitarium under the watchful and authoritative eye of physician Henry Foster (Adams, 1984). Clifton Springs Sanitarium, progressive for its time in offering homeopathic medicine and hydrotherapy, identified occupational therapy as a mode of treatment as early as 1914, three years prior to the incorporation in 1917 of occupational therapy's national society (Cayleff, 1987; Gevitz, 1988; Gifford, 1984, 2000; Starr, 1982). Occupational therapy work at Foster's hospital grew, with a full working farm, print shop, restaurant, and solarium where patients remained active under the supervision of nurses and nursing students (Adams, 1984).

In March 1917, Barton invited Thomas B. Kidner, Commissioner of Canadian Military Hospitals; Susan Johnson, of the New York Department of Charities; Dr. Dunton; Mrs. Slagle; and Isabel Newton, Barton's secretary and future wife; to a meeting at Consolation House. This group formed the National Society for the Promotion of Occupational Therapy (NSPOT). Dunton, Johnson, Slagle, Barton, and Tracy, absent at the Clifton Springs meeting, formed NSPOT's incorporating body of directors (Dunton, 1947).

From its inception, occupational therapy espoused scientific knowledge, as stated in its purpose: "for the advancement of occupation as a therapeutic measure; for the study of the effect of occupation upon the human being; and for the scientific dispensation of this knowledge" (AOTA, 1967, p. 4). Building a new national organization, Barton served as NSPOT's president, Slagle was vice president, Dunton was treasurer, and Newton was secretary. Six months after incorporation, membership had grown from 7 to 40.

Eleanor Clarke Slagle, described as "the Jane Addams of occupational therapy" for her reform efforts and doing good works similar to other women of her class, came from an influential wealthy New York family (Cromwell, 1977; Quiroga, 1995, p. 35). Close to her brother Congressman John Clarke of New York, Mrs. Slagle shared the altruistic upper class white custom that work and money was best employed for society's betterment (Veblen, 1899/1994).

Bringing this tone to occupational therapy influenced occupational therapy's recruitment for proper white, "young ladies," who would maintain these worthy and privileged values. Perhaps unintended, these potentially biased roots also promoted a white occupational therapy, limiting racial and class diversity. What is lacking in historical literature is a comprehensive discussion about the effects of class and gender on occupational therapy professionalization (Bing, 1995; Colman, 1984; Dunton, 1950; Litterst, 1992; Quiroga, 1995; Schwartz, 1992a, 1992b).

Slagle, NSPOT's first vice president, responding to early membership needs, gathered correspondence from new therapists describing early practice hurdles. Having no standardized job descriptions or wage criteria, 1920s therapists worked long hours and days having alternate Sundays off. With salaries around $40 a month, occupational therapists, besides being patient care givers, doubled as hospital hostesses arranging flowers and dances, familiar tasks for young women of society, but professionally questionable. In nursing's shadow and with skills that were not well-employed, therapists stayed the course, continuing to do good works, and slowly increasing in numbers.

World War I marked a new opportunity for the fledgling occupation. Dunton, Tracy, and Slagle approached the armed forces, initially meeting military physician opposition. A breakthrough came in 1918, when Surgeon General Gorgas of the United States Army authorized the appointment of the war "reconstruction aid" to serve in Army hospitals. Initially, six therapists served at European military hospitals. General Pershing requested an additional 200 aides. This group trained at Bloomingdale Hospital, now New York Hospital in White Plains, New York. Because these aides were popular, Pershing ordered 1,000 more aides immediately, with another 4,000 in six months. They worked with shell-shocked and crippled soldiers. Additional aides, recruited from the social work and library science professions, completed a six-week training course developed by Dunton and Slagle. Short training courses flourished in Boston, Philadelphia, St. Louis, and Baltimore. The crisis during the war was deemed a "manpower shortage." At the war's end, the next problem was what to do with all these aides. Between World War I and World War II there was a slow growth period for occupational therapy, and many changes related to organizational restructuring (Kahmann & West, 1947).

Physician Herbert Hall, NSPOT president, instituted a national society name change to the American Occupational Therapy Association (AOTA) in 1921. Two years later, Eleanor Clarke Slagle became the first executive secretary, with a title change to Executive Director of AOTA, the organization's first paid position. Mrs. Slagle held the position until 1938. The number of occupational therapy's educational programs grew during Slagle's administration. In 1935, AOTA, in collaboration with the American Medical Association (AMA), set standards for four acceptable university programs located in Boston, Milwaukee, Philadelphia, and St. Louis. A fifth program was approved the following year in Kalamazoo. These schools became the training sites for the early community of therapists. The Boston and Philadelphia Schools carried much social status and were partly supported by old eastern money and tradition. The early 1930s marked occupational therapy's shift from the non-professional training aide-level therapist to the college-educated therapist. Some attempts to change the level of education were delayed during the Great Depression, when occupational therapy's growth remained at a steady state.

After the depression years and as in World War I, occupational therapy prospered during World War II. Between 1941 and 1943 AOTA worked with the National Research Council to assist Army and Navy medical departments in assessing military needs. This military link proved significant to the community of therapists, some of whom chose military service.

Lieutenant Colonel Walter Barton, an assistant in the Neuropsychiatry Consultants Division, Office of the Surgeon General, Washington, DC, supported professional standards for occupational therapists in the War Department as part of the Civil Service Division in 1943. Qualifying therapists being graduated from educational programs which were accredited by the Council on Medical Education of the American Medical Association (CME–AMA) and who had attained national AOTA registration, were military officers.

Civilian registered occupational therapists in the army had to complete an additional two weeks training course sponsored at three centers in 1944: Lovell General Hospital, in Massachusetts, Lawson General Hospital in Georgia, or Letterman General Hospital in California. Mrs. Winifred C. Kahmann, Director of Occupational and Physical Therapy, Indiana University Medical Center, and Chairman of the War Service Committee of AOTA, was appointed Chief of the Occupational Therapy Branch of the Reconditioning Division of the Office of the Surgeon General, United States Army, November 18, 1943. Kahmann, rising to the rank of AOTA president four years later, is vividly remembered in some of the therapists' accounts later in this work.

Echoing World War I mobilization, once again occupational therapy quickly met war needs. Initially 43 occupational therapists served in 30 Army hospitals, which had an immediate need for 300 therapists, and an estimated need of 1,000 additional army occupational therapists. War Emergency Courses started July 1943, and by July 1945, 21 courses existed with a total enrollment of 665 students. Expanding occupational therapy educational programs such as the Boston School of Occupational Therapy, Columbia University, the Philadelphia School, the Richmond Professional Institute of the College of William and Mary, the University of Illinois, Milwaukee–Downer College, Mills College, and the University of Southern California offered war emergency courses. When compared with World War I, in which occupational therapists fell under a sub professional classification—the heading of Arts and Crafts and Trades Industries—the World War II therapist was classified as a scientific, or professional position under the Starnes–Schrugham Act, P.L. 359 Veterans Preference Act of 1944, marking occupational therapy's professionalization and road toward science.

Military occupational therapists such as Kahmann, her assistants Wilma West and Mary Reilly, and Ruth Robinson, later entered the innermost ranks of the community of therapists. Leaders Kahmann (1947–1952), West (1961–1964), and Robinson (1955–1958) served as AOTA presidents. Scholar Reilly took an academic career path at the University of Southern California. Post World War II occupational therapy boomed, having gained war year visibility, and a part of postwar medical rehabilitation efforts (Kahmann & West, 1947).

A Dynamic 30 Years

Occupational therapy's dynamic thirty years, 1950 until 1980, initially riding a postwar boom, were directed by proven leaders. AOTA's first occupational therapist Executive Director Wilma L. West, and first occupational therapist President Winifred Kahmann, continued their wartime working collaboration and led the organization in 1950. West had a talent for finding money for occupational therapy and new platforms. Politically savvy, she was a foremost member of the profession's "old girls' club," and a leading inner circle member of the community of therapists, along with Kahmann and the socially placed Helen Willard, as well as Beatrice Wade. These women, rising to the highest ranks of occupational therapy organizational authority, made decisions that blazed new trails (West, 1979).

West, called Willie by her peers, was "a friend" (reflecting inner circle) to the ten therapists described in this work, providing avenues, introductions, networking, peer decision-making, resources, and opportunities. Florence Cromwell remembered West, relaying:

> We know her so very well. West and Welles sat next to each other all through OT school, because you always sat alphabetically. But Willie was such an astute strategist. She knew lots of things that needed to be done. And she didn't interfere with things that you were doing, but she made good suggestions." (Cromwell/Peters oral history, April 28–29, 2003, lines 2,655–2,664)

Inner circle occupational therapy "friendship" meant career growth, collegial affirmation, mentorship, and trust when working together to strengthen occupational therapy's position in society. Carlotta Welles echoes these sentiments: "But we're very proud of OT, very proud of a lot of our colleagues, many good friends among them" (Cromwell/Peters oral history, April 28–29, 2003, lines 5377–5379). A politically savvy individual, West made things happen, prioritizing professional autonomy, education, and research as occupational therapy's key to future development. She understood placement, people and connections.

West took the executive director position in 1948, at a time when occupational therapy had just surfaced from a precarious physical medicine dispute. Physiatry, a new branch of medicine, wanted to subsume occupational therapy to gain political strength in a medical climate that deemed it a low priority practice area (West, 1992). Occupational therapy's fight for autonomy with physical medicine was one example of future turf disputes navigated by West and her peers Willard and Wade.

In 1965, the AOTF, a non-profit organization "dedicated to expanding the body of knowledge for occupational therapy, and advancing practice of the highest quality," was founded (AOTF, 2000a, p. 6; Yerxa, 1967b) with

West's support. Founding members Brunyate, Crampton, and Fidler described AOTF's mission as developing an occupational therapy think tank to advance occupational therapy's scientific body of knowledge. The foundation, initially lacking funds, formed as a separate non-profit agency from AOTA that could raise tax-deductible financial donations. Though the arrangement was not formalized, in practice, the foundation was kept afloat by AOTA for its first 10 years. West played a prominent role in the burgeoning foundation, particularly because she came from AOTA leadership positions. West, supporting research, facilitated the foundation's mission to formalize and promote scientific research for the profession.

Secondly, under AOTA President Ruth Brunyate's (later Wiemer) leadership from 1964 until 1967, occupational therapy's membership had more of a voice through the association's newly created Delegate Assembly. Wiemer and West were close colleagues. The Delegate Assembly was AOTA's elected representative body noted for bringing in a grass roots membership voice, which also mirrored the larger 1960s and 1970s social activism. West, working on the foundation side, and Wiemer's successor AOTA President Florence Cromwell guided the Delegate Assembly. In 1972 the Delegate Assembly adopted a motion that 2% of membership fees would go to AOTF. It was an unprecedented move and the entire membership now supported the foundation, expanding occupational therapy's research interests (AOTF, 1975, 2000b; Jones, 1992). During her term, Cromwell moved the association's national headquarters from New York City to the Washington, DC area, giving the profession more proximity to federal contacts.

Newly aware of a national pulse, some members of AOTA, stimulated by the civil rights and women's rights movements in the 1960s, and discussed in later chapters, changed occupational therapy. Platforming human rights awareness in the daily news and mass media, minority voices, including women and people of color, became more prominent. Integration for all people, including people with disabilities, took center stage formalizing into a disabilities movement that occupational therapists joined.

Affecting occupational therapy on multiple fronts, this white, middle class, health profession lacked racial, class, and gender diversity during 1950 to 1980. Started as a wealthy, white, philanthropic community of women doing good works for the needy, occupational therapy saw changes in the post-Cold War period related to race, class, and gender. Small numbers of men and women of color were starting to change occupational therapy's founding years' landscape. Sparse in numbers, however, these few men, typically white, and some black women rose to leadership positions, bucking the conventional 30-year occupational therapy tradition. A change from occupational therapy's white Anglo-Saxon roots was not to come quickly, because the profession still lacked representation from other ethnic minority cohorts, or foreign-born therapists, except for white female British and Canadian therapists who blended in well.

Adding to this mix, occupational therapy leaders' private lifestyles influenced the profession. Though the facts were generally not discussed, these women often had same sex housemates, and some were publicly linked romantically. These relationships served to create a close-knit group that appeared to help in positioning the brightest into the invited inner circle of the community of therapists. Occupational therapists often partnered with occupational and physical therapists. Parallel to these lesbian groupings there were rumored concerns about gay men entering the ranks and earning clinical and academic occupational therapy positions. What effect did these lifestyles have for occupational therapy's road to professionalism and science?

Such relationships, often seen as taboo, existed in a parallel fashion with a basic conservative bent in the profession, particularly in the 1950s and lingering into the 1960s and 1970s. Understandable at the time, not mixing public and private lives seemed antithetical to how occupational therapy's core group functioned. Occupational therapy leaders operated politically using a powerful women's network and placing their "friends" in prime decision making positions, often blurring public and private lines. Ultimately, how someone entered the inner or outer occupational therapy circles in the community of therapists rested upon occupational therapy pedigree, connections, and brains (Abbott, 1988).

Reflecting a changing society relating to civil rights and women's issues, occupational therapy's second 30 years demanded re-examination and redefinition. Cold War competition for expert scientific knowledge led the race to space in the 1960s, and this race was a male-dominated frontier. Open to new ideas, progressive Americans began rejecting conservatism and bureaucracy while accepting activism that carried through the 1970s (May, 1988). A new liberal social platform afforded a new podium for women. The 1960s women's movement, a human rights social movement aiming for empowerment and equality for all women in this country, gave women avenues to discuss role changes and conflicts that meshed with new beliefs and career opportunities (Friedan, 1963). While other women were seeking authority in male-dominated professions, women occupational therapists secured power internally. Women's rights arguments fell on neutral occupational therapy ears at times, to the concern of some feminist therapists like Gilfoyle (1984), Yerxa (1975), Johnson (1973), and Johnson et al. (1972). In all fairness, considering that women held the authority positions in occupational therapy and had their voices heard internally, some feminist frontiers were not groundbreaking for this female profession. Leading occupational therapists like West, Wade, Cromwell, and Fidler already knew how to play at a man's game. Male occupational therapists then and now remain a minority cohort. Female occupational therapists joined other white, educated women developing careers when many women still stayed at home to raise families.

President John F. Kennedy shifted the nation's attention to science and the race to space in the 1960s. Health care gained a new financial footing in this environment, providing avenues for expansion and research. Capable occupational therapists, newly capturing research dollars, saw scientific research as a worthy endeavor in identifying the need for a new professional legitimacy. Science, taking hold in the 1960s and even more prominently in the 1970s, meant professional legitimacy.

Debate About Scientific Inquiry

A debate currently exists about scientific inquiry's place in occupational therapy. There is little wonder why this complex discussion is ongoing today and why it existed historically. Epistemologists differ when they discuss a profession's knowledge and its relationship to rewards, power, and purpose (Elgin, 1998).

Those discussing scientific inquiry add to the complexity of the matter by arguing the merits of basic or applied research and which approach best addresses the needs of the profession (Christiansen, 1981; Duchek & Thessing, 1996; Kielhofner, 1997; Ottenbacher, 1992; Yerxa, 1987). Critics state that selective debates about research methodologies detract us from progressing as a profession and becoming competent scholars (Abreu, Peloquin, & Ottenbacher, 1998; Mosey, 1993; Ottenbacher, 1992).

Some occupational therapy scholars criticize the merits of traditional science as being too "reductionistic" of a view of practice, one that divides phenomena into "diagnostic" component parts. In contrast, other scholars are suggesting movement in a new direction, toward an individualistic, phenomenological, epistemological approach that includes life histories and narratives, ethnographic research, historical and philosophical inquiry (Burke, 1996; Parham, 1998; Yerxa, 1998, 1995, 1992). Supporters of this view are concerned that quantitative, rather than qualitative, research studies are typically funded, thereby shaping occupational therapy knowledge that misrepresents the practice as a whole (Burke, 1996; Duchek & Thessing, 1996).

Generally overlooked in today's discussions is an understanding of past events that have led to the present debates about occupational therapy's supporting body of knowledge. More specifically, present day debates have not been compared to a time in the profession's history when scientific inquiry was emerging. Much of the discussion among occupational therapy scholars is about varying epistemological approaches to practice, or the nature, scope, and utility of occupational therapy knowledge. Generally, today's practitioner recognizes terms like "best practice," "outcome studies research," and "evidence-based" rather than epistemological approaches to practice. These label differences, which carry varying meanings, add to today's confusion. A similar epistemological discussion originated 50 years ago which was described as a need for research. Occupational therapists have not compared these two periods of occupational therapy history; however, I believe this link is central to a better understanding of occupational therapy's current status as a profession and its supporting body of knowledge.

Notable discussion about the importance of scientific inquiry did not occur until the 1950s, following a national consciousness about technological advances initiated during the war years (Custard, 1998). During the 1950s and 1960s, progressive occupational therapists adopted a view that a more scientific approach to practice was congruent with a national enthusiasm for traditional scientific models (Hollis, 1979; Kuhn, 1970). On the heels of World War II, when technology had become key to economic and military power, scientific knowledge was lauded as the future of the nation. By the 1950s and in the following decades, science moved beyond the confines of the military, universities, and government agencies to every aspect of American life, including health care (Dickson, 1988).

In the 1980s, a new generation of occupational therapists discussed paradigm shifts in the profession's knowledge base (Clark, 1979; Kielhofner, 1980; Kielhofner & Burke, 1983; Rogers, 1982, 1983; Scardina, 1981). Shifts in paradigms meant a questioning of scientific practice and application, theory development, and previous research models (Kuhn, 1970). Occupational therapists supporting this new thinking proclaimed a narrow or reductionistic view of science was too limiting. Thus an important debate began in occupational therapy, and it continues to this day concerning various epistemological approaches to practice.

Epistemological Orientations to Practice

Spending a 40-year career studying occupational therapy's knowledge base, Anne Cronin Mosey is well placed in occupational therapy's scientific inquiry debate.[3] Mosey's (1996) taxonomy describes how occupational therapy created and used its knowledge. According to Mosey, in its 80-year history, occupational therapy has had four epistemological orientations to practice: traditional, disciplinal, neopositivistic, and phenomenological.[4] All epistemological orientations can be seen simultaneously in occupational therapy practice today. Mosey believes the disciplinal and neopositivistic orientations to practice developed simultaneously, providing occupational therapy's science-based supporting body of knowledge. I believe the traditional, disciplinal, and neopositivistic orientations to practice coincided with occupational therapy's evolution to a science-based profession between 1950 and 1980. In contrast, the phenomenological orientation to practice has been more prevalent since 1990. What is relevant from a historical perspective is an investigation of why occupational therapy scholars embraced different epistemological orientations to practice during different times in the profession's history.

This debate suggests the direction of the profession and the meaning of its supporting body of knowledge. The outcome of the debate is still unknown. Related to the debate about scientific inquiry, and historically significant, the occupational therapy body of knowledge did not evolve in a vacuum. A driving question is how and with whom did occupational therapists interact? I have selected Andrew Abbott's (1988) conceptual framework, "The System of Professions" to explore this question further arguing that occupational therapy did not evolve alone or in isolation. The community of therapists moved the profession forward, responding to historical, cultural, and societal needs and opportunities.

Conceptual Framework: The System of Professions

The System of Professions, a theoretical model, describes how professions function and evolve, act and react to historical events, in an interacting or ecological system (Abbott, 1988). Structurally, the System of Professions is a three-level model labeled *social forces, system of professions,* and *differentiation*, describing how professions create their work and evolve a body of knowledge (see Figure 1).

Social forces, at the top of the hierarchy, are external agents like client needs and funding policies, influencing change in the individual profession. The *system of professions*, the center level of the hierarchy, describes how persons in professions interact, gaining jurisdiction that initiates a chain effect or reaction in the system. Finally, the predominant profession, gaining jurisdiction or political power, remains the most viable in a competitive field (see Figure 2).

Differentiation occurs at the lowest level of the hierarchy, when the individual profession responds to internal or external events that demand action. Post 1950s, occupational therapists differentiated their work in various ways, including creating an abstract body of knowledge, stratifying educational requirements, and defining different practice specialties. Overall,

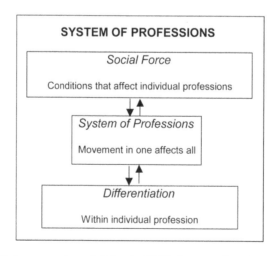

FIGURE 1 Interpretation of Abbott's (1988) System of Professions model.

1. New groups emerge by filling a vacancy or through interprofessional contests.

2. Forces within professions strengthen or weaken jurisdiction, including developing new knowledge.

3. Disturbances in the system propagate.

4. Strategies to move through the system disturbances (creating and absorbing tasks and groups, changing the level of abstract knowledge).

5. Further change in jurisdictional ties occurs internally and externally.

6. Homeostasis of forces occurs.

7. A seizure of vacant jurisdiction occur.

8. A profession makes a new claim to gain jurisdictions.

FIGURE 2 Professional jurisdictions: Chain of effects.

change or movement in one profession affects all other professions involved in the System of Professions through various internal and external means.[5] Ultimately, the more viable occupational therapy became, the more it could answer specific societal needs.

Significant to occupational therapy, the System of Professions portrays how professional paths are created, changed, eliminated and maintained (Clarke, 1989; Perkins, 1991; Turner, 1989). It also brings into the forefront the importance of knowledge development to occupational therapy. I agree with critics who portray the model as overburdened with concepts that confuse the reader. Secondly, there is so much emphasis on the sociology of the division of labor that some question whether this is a model well-suited for the study of the history of professions (Di Maggio, 1989; Turner, 1989). Taking into consideration strengths and weaknesses, this conceptual framework can be helpful in understanding occupational therapy's second 30-year professionalization process. Adding texture and insight to this study, and understanding the profession, in addition to the conceptual model, is my own experience as an occupational therapist.

ABOUT THE AUTHOR/RESEARCHER

My professional career commenced in the early 1980s, representing the years immediately following this study. I began studying occupational therapy's professionalization as a female professional during my master's studies in the 1980s. As an occupational therapy doctoral student at New York University in the 1990s, I was particularly drawn to Mosey's work while I was her student and was learning more about the debates surrounding scientific inquiry. I thought current debates about scientific inquiry were limited without understanding past trends and anomalies in occupational therapy history.

Having more than 20 years of experience as an occupational therapist, my own entrance into the profession coincided with the professional careers of those I studied. I knew some of the past AOTA presidents' work while they were in office, and recognized others' names or reputations. This proved an interesting conjunction when I gathered oral histories or reviewed documents because, in some cases, the information before me was part of my own professional history and memories. Coincidentally, or perhaps not, I have also been a student of some of the occupational therapy scholars mentioned in these pages, namely Lela Augustus Llorens (Peters, 1987) and Anne Cronin Mosey, giving me prior exposure to their thinking and mentoring. I also have held elected and appointed volunteer leadership positions in AOTA and AOTF, providing me with a working relationship and/or introductions to some of the leaders I interviewed. This said, I intended to give as fair and accurate a description of past events as possible, while knowing the potential pitfalls that could come through my telling their stories.

I discussed occupational therapy's epistemological foundations with various scholars over the years, some included in these pages, and others not, adding to my curiosity about these foundations. These occupational therapists helped shape my thinking about the need to study and record occupational therapy's professional progress, building a supporting body of knowledge. I view these discussions as assets, rather than limitations, in helping me to understand occupational therapy's history.

I have also taught occupational therapy's history and application to university students, who challenged my views about the meaning of history in today's practice environment. Skillfully, students argued that occupational therapy's past practice was obsolete in light of today's standards. Their arguments cite important new technological advances, but overlook how occupational therapists made professional advances in the context of their own times. Lessons, I believe, can be learned from history. Understanding how opportunities are gained and lost is an important history lesson when applied to today's professional dilemmas. These discussions and experiences gave me opportunities to question my own views. Grasping for a deeper understanding and recapturing occupational therapy's past brings meaning to the present.

Rudimentary discussions about occupational therapy research and scientific approaches to practice began earlier then the time frame of this study. Occupational therapy's second 30 years however, marked a time when practice became theoretically grounded. Finally having a language and means to articulate what they were doing and why it was working, therapists more skillfully explained their treatment strategies to patients, family members, and other professionals. This is not meant to discredit occupational therapy practice prior to 1950, its worth, or value. What this does bring to light is a level of sophistication and evolution beyond a traditional epistemological approach which uses trial and error or apprenticeship methods. It is also erroneous to think that theory development dominated in the 1950s; few in fact spoke in such terms. It was a gradual process that became more evident in the 1970s.

Addressing potential bias, I acknowledge my standing as an occupational therapist studying occupational therapy. Particularly, I must consider a historical debate about objectivity and merit when a researcher is part of the culture being studied (Ritchie, 1995). Undeniably, I am subject to a biased aggrandizement of my own profession, and must remain vigilant to avoid this pitfall. I also appreciate that to a larger reading audience, occupational therapy and the names in these pages known to occupational therapists, are of little consequence or unfamiliar. What is important is the telling of one small health profession's struggle to remain viable and grow in scholarship, led by a group of women at a time when this country was open to scientific debate. Secondly, it was a time when women made their stance known, to gain an independent authority as professionals, which has meaning beyond occupational therapy.

All researchers come with their own history and biases that can inform or hinder the outcome of an argument. I clearly state a deep respect for the legacy and work the occupational therapists participating in this study represent. I knew or had known about most of these people prior to this work. I didn't, however, know the extent of their work, either individually or collectively, or the context of their times until I immersed myself in the work.

Mindful of these issues, I challenged myself to understand these therapists as people, rather than professional symbols or icons, in order to remain fair to them and occupational therapy history. This dilemma illustrates the paradoxical complexity I faced, being an occupational therapist studying occupational therapy. On one hand, I entered the work understanding occupational culture, stated and coded language, and values. On the other hand, I struggled in the search for research objectivity, asking myself how someone outside of occupational therapy would view this information?

Fortuitously, being an occupational therapist provided me access. Certain participants stated their willingness to pass the torch or entrust information to a member of their profession. My experiences varied when I gathered oral histories. In some cases I was interviewed about my own professional background and history, unlocking a mutual sharing, providing a testing ground, or facilitating an authenticity of commitment. Each oral history entered was a shared partnership.

Conversely, my status as an occupational therapist worked against me if participants created filters to screen information about a mutual profession. Blatant candor meant demystifying some occupational therapists in new ways, or testing previously taboo waters. If I were not an occupational therapist, would I be in a better position to challenge a tradition I wasn't a part of? A valid consideration and limitation in any oral history work is informants' creating walls, consciously or unconsciously, to glorify their professional and private past. Once again I realize my burden is to present a complete and fair occupational therapy history taking into consideration people's lives and the complexities of their time.

SECTION II: THE STUDY

Study Design

Using a social historical research methodology, I studied how and why occupational therapy scholars and leaders, as a cohort, promoted scientific inquiry (Appleby, Hunt, & Jacob, 1994).[6] Besides seeing this community of therapists as a study unit, I realized that the crucial data came from their individual oral histories, which provided salient information and intimate details. Their words and reflections animated occupational therapy's second 30 years beyond existing documents. I then started reconstructing a more extensive historical account about this community and the people who changed occupational therapy.

Because of my historical approach, I tried locating myself in occupational therapy in the 1950s, recreating time, place, context, climate, and consciousness (Bloch, 1953; Gottshalk, 1969). Spending months and eventually years immersing myself in occupational therapy's past, I read materials and listened to therapists speak about the state of the profession as they saw it. The more than 6 months I spent gathering oral histories proved unexpectedly profound. Rather than solely gathering research information, I heard life stories and learned life lessons. I listened, read, and contemplated how these individuals navigated occupational therapy and their lives, seeking back stories, and the whys behind their actions.

After each taping, I spent time reflecting on their careers and life-path choices and tried to walk in their shoes. Totally unexpectedly, I can describe visceral life-affirming experiences after spending time with these people. I found them realistic, proud, blunt, and strongly committed to a better occupational therapy. Frequently contacting my dissertation chair and other professors while traveling throughout the United States doing my fieldwork, I spilled out this wonderment. Writing now, I think not only about these therapists, but the therapists I wasn't able to tape. How would the weaving have changed if I had heard both insider and outsider stories?

I compared my own career steps, trying to understand the community of therapists' choices and to unravel their narratives. I will refrain from factoring in my own story when recounting theirs,' except in cases where our histories collide. I think choosing to write in the first person illustrates my immersion into their culture and intimate experiences. Clearly I wasn't a member, rather a keen observer representing the next generation of occupational therapists. Nonetheless, I took a researcher's stance, knowing that distance and objectivity needed to remain a cornerstone when analyzing history.

There is also a personal element that goes into writing about their accounts that reaches beyond my expectations that touched and challenged me while I was doing this work. Whether it was the power of their words, their spirit, or their personalities, stepping into their lives as they opened their homes to me proved provocative. I continued to wonder why this particular cohort became the theory developers and tradition breakers, exploring common threads and differences. They varied in ethnic backgrounds, socio-economic roots, and lifestyles, but they commonly believed occupational therapy to be a worthy profession and invested their talents in it. Intelligent and gifted, they had other career options, but they consciously chose and stayed with occupational therapy. Why?

The months and hours I spent transcribing oral histories, reviewing information, hearing it over and over, helped me to recapture the intensity and strength of affect, appreciating new passages that became part of a whole or arose from a group of interviews. Parallels arose, and it wasn't uncommon for different leaders to tell similar stories. That was surprising considering how individualistic each person was. Spurred on by their words, I was able to relive and somehow step back into their pasts better informed. I asked myself questions, new and ongoing, that arose from the information I gathered. Each transcript drew me back to the fieldwork experience.

During fieldwork, I spent hours and days entering their homes, and also the current lives of these therapists. I was graciously welcomed as an intellectual peer by many, treated like an old or new friend, or someone to mentor, and during our time together was able to characteristically travel to an intellectual debate about occupational therapy's past, present, and future. I sat in their living rooms, kitchens, dining rooms, and family rooms listening to their words. I toured their homes, gardens, and experienced their larger communities with them across the United States. On one occasion I left with a bag full of lemons Carlotta Welles and I picked together, returning East carrying sweet memories. I learned later from her peers that I entered a friendship ritual known to them for years. I met therapists' family members and friends, and played with their cherished pets who managed to make their voices known during taping. Taking on their daily rhythms in contrasting landscapes, I gathered oral histories in northeastern cities, like Boston, New York, and Washington, DC, I traveled to tropical Florida, the Texas Gulf Coast, and shared expansive Colorado, California, and Texas vistas. I spent time in urban, suburban, and rural settings, seeing stately Civil War mansions on Maryland's Eastern Shore, walking Florida beaches, and spending a family outing where I saw my first wild elk in Estes Park, Colorado. I drove miles and miles of the great California desert and Sierra foothills to spend time at the mountaintop home of one occupational therapy scholar, viewing a sunset over a tranquil backyard ravine of another, and visiting architecturally interesting Scripps College with a 1930s alumna. This contrasted to a fast-paced Washington, DC interview and archival visit.

I learned about these therapists' families, viewed their children's cherished trophies, examined art collections, family heirlooms, and deceased parents' pictures. From all these rich materials, I learned who these people are, and about their roots, values, and grounding. I also enjoyed hours of formal and informal conversation over meals, cups of coffee, tea, and cocktails and toasting a grand profession's past and future, as well as our own. These were times when we shared laughter, hope, and when therapists remembered fondly, and with some tearful grief, the times and people lost. I was honored to be privy to such open sharing, and accepted their kindness as our lives converged. While doing fieldwork, attending occupational therapy national conferences, and speaking informally to the community of therapists' peers and my peers through the years, I overwhelmingly experienced support and thanks for taking on this historical task deemed necessary and important. Though I was not swept into a mission or calling, I learned that occupational therapy history needs to be recorded for current and future generations.

I share my personal account of doing this work not only to inform readers about how I gathered and experienced a living history, but to illustrate my personal involvement in the subject matter. There is a fine line between cultural immersion and subjectivity. While doing the work, I continually examined my own objectivity, and engaged in a personal struggle. While listening to the oral histories I wondered how my questions or non-verbal interactions may have influenced an oral history direction, a shift in thought, or an outcome. Although I stated at the start of each taping that I was there to hear the memoirist's reflections, expecting each telling to be unique, I doubted my own method and wondered about my questioning style and the questions themselves. Did my questions cut off a thought prematurely, or derail the memoirist's thinking in any way? Were they leading, or biased, or did I find out what I really needed to know? This became the subject of many journal entries throughout the year.

In listening to the tapes, I continued to study the flow and direction, asking myself what the hidden story was. Here I relied on print sources to compare and verify information. Adding to the complexity of my personal influence on the data was the potential bias in how I gathered the material. Each therapist's story represented one person's opinion and experience, and was open to questioning. Time was a factor, and some childhood memories of events that had occurred 50–70 years ago were, undoubtedly, not always accurate. Frequently, therapists remembered career vignettes but not specific dates. I found that piecing together enough of a story with written documents, another person's account, or published articles solved many puzzles. In remembering their pasts, I questioned why they remembered certain vignettes and not others? What were these therapists really saying when recounting this story?

Similarly, the remaining archival documents had their own challenges, giving only a partial historical picture. Many documents were discarded when AOTA relocated from New York to the Washington, DC area in the 1970s. The profession's archival library also relocated. First organized and housed at the University of Texas, Galveston, Moody Library under community member and occupational therapy historian Robert K. Bing in the 1970s and 1980s, they were later relocated to the Wilma L. West Library at AOTA and AOTF's national headquarters in Bethesda, Maryland. Aware of these archival pitfalls, I asked myself why some records remained while others did not. Were documents lost, discarded purposefully, or unintentionally? Are missing documents privately stored? Lastly, I examined why I choose the documents and words I used in making my interpretations.

Understandably, most history remains subjective, and open to misinterpretation. This discipline of study requires thoughtful and painstaking rigor. The alternative is perpetuating or promulgating an incorrect, outdated explanation, analysis, or belief. My historical hunt or the art of recreating this occupational therapy history required creatively searching and evaluating multiple sources for the most accurate information. Subjectivity, sometimes viewed as a negative word, is accepted as a necessary challenge when striving for objectivity, from a historian's perspective. The challenge lies in the nature of history itself, obtaining often incomplete information from the past and making contextual judgments about the meaning, significance, and relevance of the information (Cantor & Schneider, 1967).

Doing this historical research mandated asking questions, critically examining and analyzing evidence, and finally, constructing arguments to support conclusions (Fischer, 1970; Gottshalk, 1969; Rampolla, 2001). History, as a whole, is more than the surviving records or a static chronology; it is dynamic and interactive (Kaestle, 1996). Historiography recreates a close approximation of the past from data using clear guidelines of analysis.[7] Here lies the argument for more rigorous study, and a way to more objectively evaluate this study. Reconstructing occupational therapy scholars' and leaders' personal stories required understanding relative truths, measured against informed questions and theoretical constructs, thus creating new information or paradigms.

SOURCES OF DATA

I collected data from a variety of sources: archived unpublished primary materials, published primary and secondary source materials, private papers, artifacts and photographs of individuals participating in the study, e-mail correspondence, a recorded oral history in the oral histories collection of the AOTF, oral history interviews, and New York University Occupational Therapy Department records.

Primary and secondary sources. The primary sources I selected are eyewitness accounts, papers, and books published from 1950–1980, curricula vitae, photographs, 8 mm film, awards and documents, art work, memorabilia, private papers such as family correspondence and photographs, letters and memoirs, and interviewee's published and unpublished professional articles authored throughout their careers. I reviewed all issues of the *American Journal of Occupational Therapy* (AJOT), the official publication of the AOTA, published from 1950–1980. Primary sources are materials and remaining records that convey an author or interviewee's actions, thoughts, and beliefs related directly to the events that he or she reports (Brooks, 1969; Gottshalk, 1969; Marius, 1999).

Archival materials. I mailed separate letters to the Executive Directors of AOTA and AOTF, on February 5, 2003, requesting access to the archives of both organizations housed in the Wilma L. West Library (WLW) at the AOTF. I printed the letters on New York University Occupational Therapy Departmental stationery, stating my qualifications, the nature of the study, and the types and historical time frame of materials needed. I requested no more than four months of archival access to collect data. I asked that they contact me if there were any concerns; otherwise I planned to make appointments to review the archival documents. I received confirmation in e-mail from Martha Kirkland, Executive Director of the AOTF, welcoming me to the collection, offering to help beyond a document search. I also sent a letter to the WLW archivist Mary Binderman, explaining my study. She informed me the archival collection included AOTA's and AOTF's historical records.

I reviewed confidential organizational memorandums, unpublished meeting minutes, funding reports, correspondence, workshop proceedings, grant funded research projects, organizational promotional materials, and photographs at the WLW library. To complete the document search, I gathered other information from three sources, two private collections that included professional and personal papers, and artifacts of occupational therapists Marion Crampton in Massachusetts, and Robert K. Bing, in Texas. I traveled to both states to review these collections. I gathered other primary print information from New York University's Bobst Library and the New York University Occupational Therapy Department.

The secondary sources I used, or that information supporting primary sources, included occupational therapy journal articles published in AJOT, the *Occupational Therapy Journal of Research* (OTJR), and other AOTA publications including official white papers, education bulletins, and the like published after 1980. I also reviewed pamphlets, private papers, and other source materials written, published, or dated after 1980. The secondary sources spanned a broad range of topics besides occupational therapy, such as other health care professions including medicine and nursing, the rehabilitation movement, and United States and women's history. I also gathered secondary materials at the Clifton Springs Historical Society, in Clifton Springs, New York, in November 2003.

Interviewees. I selected oral histories, or the gathering and preserving of information through recorded interviews, because they are a uniquely living form of history. Arguably valid alone, oral histories also fill in gaps in existing archival records (Oral History Association, 2001). Occupational therapists gave their in-depth oral histories which ranged from 2.5–16 hours. Eleven therapists participated between December 2002 and April 2003. A twelfth therapist participated in a pilot study in 1997. I traveled, in this order, to New York (twice), Colorado, Massachusetts, Florida, Maryland, Washington, DC, and California to collect oral histories. I selected recognized occupational therapy scholars and leaders who served in clinical, administrative, or academic positions between 1950 and 1980. For this study, occupational therapy scholars are people who have received the profession's highest scholarly award, the Eleanor Clarke Slagle lectureship, and who have had a publication record of books and/or articles in juried journals, who have had advanced academic education, and were Fellows of the AOTA. Occupational therapy leaders selected for this study received AOTA's highest service award, the Award of Merit, served either AOTA and/or AOTF in appointed or elected offices or similar volunteer positions, and were Fellows of the AOTA. These candidates also needed to be able to logically recall and recount events concerning their professional careers, which had occurred 30–50 years earlier.

I created a pool of prospective interviewees by reviewing occupational therapy journals, pamphlets, and books circa 1950 to 1980, reviewing award recipients' names, and checking AOTA minutes and committee members' names published in the AJOT. I invited selected therapists receiving the Eleanor Clarke Slagle lectureships between 1955 (first Slagle lecture) and 1984, and selected recipients of AOTA's Award of Merit between the years 1950 and 1980, to participate in this study. This pool consisted of approximately 16 living Slagle recipients, and 10 living Award of Merit recipients. Because of frail health, retirement, or professional disengagement, the pool was narrowed to a total of 8 Slagle recipients, and 4 Award of Merit recipients. Six people in the Slagle pool received both awards, earning their Awards of Merit up to 1997, reflecting a total of 10 Awards of Merit.

I invited two additional occupational therapists to participate because of their status as executive director of AOTF and director of research at AOTF. These women knew and worked closely with the community of therapists whom I studied in-depth, but were not part of the Slagle or Merit group. Their additional interviews supported and provided information which filled in historical gaps.

I mailed 12 invitational letters at staggered time periods, coordinating individual scheduling needs between November 2002 and February 2003. This number includes the executive director of AOTF and the director of research at AOTF. I introduced myself as a researcher in the letter, explained the purpose of the study, and the plan for handling of data according to New York University's Office of Sponsored Programs Committee on Activities

Involving Human Subjects and the Principles and Standards of the Oral History Association (2001).

I gathered mailing addresses through various means, including potential participants' peers and former students, the AOTF, the New York University Occupational Therapy Department alumni association, and Internet searches. When the membership division of AOTA was contacted January 28, 2003, for mailing addresses, I was informed that individual mailing addresses could not be released; however, letters could be forwarded by mailing them first to AOTA. Given time constraints, I did not use this option. The invitational letter included a copy of the oral history consent form for initial review purposes and a response form, which was to be returned to the researcher in a stamped, self-addressed envelope within a two-week time frame, indicating acceptance or refusal of the invitation to participate in the study.

The respondents could accept the invitation by mail, a collect telephone call, or e-mail. For those who did not return the response forms within the two-week period, I mailed a second letter, which was a duplicate of the first invitational letter, with an added statement that this was a follow-up from an initial mailing. This was done for three prospective participants. In two cases I made e-mail contact in lieu of a third mailing, one directly to the participants, and another to a third party, a suggested close colleague who declined the invitation for the potential participant. Of the 10 Slagle and Merit invitation letters sent, 9 therapists agreed to participate in the study. The 10th participant in this pool agreed and participated in an extensive oral history pilot study in 1997 that I conducted under faculty supervision during a historical inquiry course at New York University.

I contacted those persons who returned their response forms indicating that they agreed to participate in the study. Either by telephone or e-mail, I discussed the study, answered initial questions, and made interview appointments. I interviewed participants at their place of residence except in one case. This person was experiencing declining health during the interviewing period and needed an adapted arrangement. We agreed to my posing a few questions at a time, using the Internet, and the participant answering them as his tolerance allowed. This occurred between December 2002 and April 2003, shortly before his death in May. All paperwork relating to the study was sent and returned via postage paid priority mail. I also remained in contact with a third party, another close occupational therapy colleague living near the participant, who agreed to deliver any necessary paperwork and gave me health updates when necessary. This third person helped most notably when I hadn't heard from the participant related to brief hospitalizations.

DATA COLLECTION

My concentrated data collection spanned the period between October 2002 and April 2003, including searching occupational therapy history data, the history of professions, and women's history sources, placing emphasis on oral history and archival materials. I began studying and collecting printed materials in 1997 as a doctoral student enrolled in historical inquiry courses. During that period I reviewed 30 years of the AJOT and occupational therapy books and pamphlets published since 1950.

Primary and secondary sources. Prior to collecting oral histories, I examined materials pertinent to the interviewees published in AJOT, OTJR, occupational therapy books, and AOTA publications, including workshop proceedings and newsletters. I conducted a two-day archival search at the WLW Library in March 2003, following 7 out of the 12 interviews. Reviewing archival materials, I sometimes viewed incomplete records which skipped years at a time, or were missing document pages, but I was able to corroborate preliminary data, and reconstruct as complete a historical record as possible. Some unexpected finds included handwritten informal notes, often initialed or signed by first name only. Identifying identities, I examined handwriting samples showing full signatures on other documents, or reviewed AOTA or AOTF organizational charts from the period to acquaint myself with staff names. I adhered to all archival procedures including handling and copying documents, and maintaining file order to preserve historical integrity of sources. Note-taking procedures included identifying the archive name, group number, papers or person, series number, and date of materials reviewed (Barzun & Graff, 1970; Brooks, 1969).

I gathered and reviewed secondary sources from New York University's Bobst Library and the New York University Occupational Therapy Department. I used secondary sources to expand my understanding of primary sources and to broaden my oral history questions (Marius, 1999; Storey, 1999).

Oral histories. I conducted all of the oral history interviews. Before each oral history, I reviewed relevant primary and secondary materials in order to be well-grounded in the subjects to be discussed. I informed the interviewees about the study's goals and objectives in the invitational letter, and again at the time of the interview, inviting participant questions prior to taping. Most participants moved quickly into the interview process asking few preliminary questions; however in some cases I was interviewed about the purpose of my work, my interest in the topic, and my professional background. Some interviewees preferred a 30–40 minute informal talking period prior to taping, as compared with those who immediately engaged in the more formal process.

In order to participate in the study, I asked interviewees to sign a consent form authorizing recording of voice, name, and recollections for scholarly and educational use. All interviewees signed the consent form prior to the taping. Five out of twelve mailed the signed the sample consent and returned it to the researcher, although they were not instructed to do this.

The remaining interviewees signed the form immediately prior to the recording, in the presence of the researcher, following discussion and clarification. All interviewees allowed the use of their name and words, which added historical resonance and depth to this study, and received copies of their signed consent form.

Although they were not selected, interviewees wanting to remain anonymous could sign an attribution statement authorizing pseudonyms and allowing their identifying characteristics to be masked. I informed participants about their rights in the oral history process, such as editing and expected dissemination of all forms of the record, as stated in the Oral History consent form. All interviewees gave the researcher permission to use their names, two requested review of final quotes prior to any publication. No participants requested review of the oral history transcripts. No participants requested the tapes be destroyed at the conclusion of the study. One participant requested, in addition to placing tapes in the WLW Library of AOTA, that a second copy of the recording be deposited in the Lela A. Llorens collection at Texas Woman's University.

To give as complete a historical record as possible, I discussed interviewees' rights to respond to questions candidly, and to seal portions of the interview or to choose to remain anonymous in sensitive circumstances. When sensitive material did arise during the interview, the interviewee asked that the recording be stopped, or that certain sections of the tape not be quoted. I complied and recorded in the transcription the stopping and restarting of the tape, or transcribed and then struck out sensitive materials. I used similar strategies in handling the e-mail data gathered in the one adapted oral history.

Participants ranged in age from 63–86 years, with a couple being physically frail, which affected interview tolerance, endurance, or taping times. In all cases I individualized the recording situations. For example, some therapists preferred early morning interviews starting at 8:00 a.m., others mid-morning or evening recordings. In one situation, I interviewed two participants together at their home, over a two-day period that spanned from morning until evening with rest periods.

I used a built-in microphone microcasette recorder with a voice-operated recording component to record the interviews. I labeled and stored all tapes in a cool, dust-free environment at my home. The tapes and transcripts included the name of the interviewer and interviewee, as well as the date, place, and time of the interview. Ideally, when available, I conducted the oral histories in a quiet, distraction-free environment. Since most tapings occurred in private homes, however, everyday household sounds are recorded including ringing telephones, background television noise, dogs barking, and conversational asides with family members. I chose to continue recording through this background noise so as not to interrupt conversation or important information.

I decided that taking handwritten notes would be too distracting and arti-ficial during the interview process, although I weighed the merit of them if there were to be a taping malfunction or oversight (Brooks, 1969). When I discovered that I had missed recording a portion of an interview, as a result of unexpected tape endings, immediately following the interview I wrote notes from memory. This proved to be exceptional rather than a common occurrence.

Following each interview session I wrote reflective notes, including descriptions of the setting, the interview content, and initial impressions. In this work I created new questions that rose from the tapings. Some ques-tions led to internal intellectual dialogue, helping me form new insights or ways of thinking about the subject matter. The richest reflections came from serendipity or the unexpected information I heard, often taking me down some new roads. I finally had to let go of many paths to find a clear direction out of my maze, and to hold firm to my guiding research questions.

I transcribed the oral histories using a computer for word processing, and after each transcription process wrote reflective notes. Simultaneously, I kept a research journal log for the entire duration of the study, noting each working session, participant contacts, all e-mail correspondence with participants and

---

Oral History Guide Questions

1. How did you get interested in occupational therapy?

2. What was it like being a therapist in the (1950s, 1960s, 1970s)? Tell me about what was going on in occupational therapy?

3. What discussions or "hot topics" were you having with colleagues at that time about the state of the profession?

4. What do you consider your major contributions to the profession?

5. Tell me about your professional accomplishments and frustrations.

6. There is an assumption in the definition of occupational therapy that the profession is moving to a science base. What is your view of this? Not everyone agreed. Who were they and how were their issues being addressed? Are they still being addressed?

7. What does it mean to you for a profession to become science-based?

8. What has the profession done to make it happen or prevent it from being science-based? What was going on in the rest of the world?

9. Is there anything else you would like to say?

FIGURE 3 Oral history guide questions.

others, thoughts about the study, and other information related to the study. Creating individual therapist folders, I reviewed all reflective notes as part of data synthesis and analysis as well as other information stored. In each participant's folder I kept not only a copy of the transcripts and reflective notes, but their curricula vitae, and a collection of their publications including journal articles and book chapters. I also included secondary print sources like occupational therapy newspaper articles noting various career milestones. Therefore, each folder provided a good overview to write from.

The oral histories proved to be unique, with each memoirist telling her or his own story in spite of some of the same questions being asked. I asked similar open-ended interview questions (see Figure 3), that I created and considered a general oral history guide (Polit & Hungler, 1995; Tuchman, 1981).

These questions stimulated discussion about the interviewee's experience as a scholar and leader. I augmented and individualized questions, taking into consideration each therapist's particular contributions to occupational therapy.[8]

DATA ANALYSIS

Data analysis involved collecting sources, examining them for genuineness, extracting credible information, and weaving them together into a plausible, coherent story that makes sense when contextualized with other analyses (Barzun & Graff, 1970; Gottschalk, 1969). Simply stated, I studied sources, compared them to a theoretical framework, and created an argument. This questioning process became an integral part of assessing external and internal criticism.

Because documents tell only parts of stories, and people giving oral histories can miss details through blurred memory or fabrication, I questioned the data open-mindedly (Barzun & Graff, 1970). To verify sources, I questioned the informers during the interview or in some cases after, through follow-up telephone calls or e-mail correspondence. I continually weighed oral data against printed sources, and questioned documents against other primary and secondary documents. When possible, I asked those familiar with the sources or particular situations to verify stories. Typically, other therapists in the community of therapists shared mutual experiences that provided overlapping reminiscences about the same events. Occupational therapy professors at New York University, who were able to give first-person accounts, also proved reliable sources when assessing information.

I spoke informally to the participants' colleagues over a three-day period at the AOTA national conference in Washington, DC in June 2003 about their reminiscences. Many offered additional anecdotal information about those interviewed or about deceased leaders that deepened my understanding. These occupational therapists stated their willingness to help me gather additional data if needed, or suggested other people to interview.

Although many of these ideas are worthy of future study, I found myself at a point of information saturation at times.

Analyzing the oral history texts, I formatted the page using a half page vertical margin. Using this space, I wrote handwritten notes to identify themes or key passages. I color-coded oral history texts, assigning different colors to different participants, that simplified identification and sorting of data. I began a process of sorting information according to the research questions and theoretical framework guiding this study. This proved a three-step weeding process, sifting through nearly 1000 transcript pages. First I sought broad topics, like research, theory, or political factors. I found the most significant oral history passages in my second data review and managed to collapse categories. Prior to a third review, I met with my dissertation chair and discussed emerging themes and categories. During this important meeting we discussed the data that most answered my research questions.

Text analysis methods included deconstructing words to compare what is stated with the intended meaning of the words, assessing potential missing information, establishing patterns to interpret themes, and identifying emotionally charged passages following speech idiosyncrasies such as pauses, or repeated phrases (Appleby, Hunt & Jacob, 1994; Cantor & Schneider, 1967; Cohen, 1994; Frisch, 1990; Ritchie, 1995; Spradley, 1979; Vansina, 1985, Wolcott, 2001).

I sorted documents, grouping them according to those authored by the community of interviewed therapists, with each participant having a separate folder. These folders eventually led to each therapist's master folder which was previously described. Similar to the oral history transcripts, I sorted these documents according to research questions and the theoretical framework, thus creating a chapter structure. I generally categorized documents as "community of therapists," organizational (AOTA/AOTF or other), and occupational therapy theory development.

External and Internal Criticism

External criticism questions the authenticity of the document, whereas internal criticism evaluates the worth of the evidence (Polit & Hunger, 1995). I assessed genuineness (external criticism) of print source materials, evaluating document genuineness via the age and color of the paper and print; location, whether archival, private collections, or library collections; and evaluating any discrepancies if there was more than one version of the same document (Barzun & Graff, 1970; Gottschalk, 1969). I discovered that unofficial handwritten notes and minutes taken at various meetings also helped to verify official documents. I thank Marion Crampton for sharing her private papers, particularly those relating to her role as founding Secretary of the AOTF. Former AOTA President Robert K. Bing, known as a "pack rat" historian, proved a gold mine, too. His private papers, including detailed handwritten notes similarly proved valuable when assessing document genuineness and credibility. I also thank former AOTA President Ruth Weimer for her private notes and AOTA conference information from her presidential years in the late 1960s.

I assessed the credibility (internal criticism) of print source materials, questioning the historical context in which the source was written, the intended audience, the purpose of the document, and potential bias (Rampolla, 2001). I assessed the reliability and validity of the oral histories, questioning information credibility, whether the information was factual or judgmental, the emotional tone, and the relationship of oral information to existing documents (Marius, 1999).

When reviewing audiotapes and transcripts, I kept a handwritten journal of thoughts and reflections questioning the material. I did not discover any internal or external authenticity problems in print sources. I did discover some inconsistencies in oral histories related to historical dates, and remembering which particular individuals attended various meetings. This was expected, given differences in eyewitness accounts, and that therapists reminisced about events occurring 30–50 years earlier. I was able to clarify all inconsistencies by reviewing print sources, or asking a third person for additional information.

Significant to external and internal criticism, Kaestle (1996) argues that establishing standards of evidence is difficult in historical inquiry because there are too many anomalies and discrepancies in data. A solution I used is framing the historical question in a way that creates a dialog between the theory and source materials. To explore this further and best use theoretical materials as intended, I contacted Dr. Andrew Abbott, at the University of Illinois, Chicago, about the System of Professions for feedback and guidance. Dr. Abbott responded via e-mail on February 19, 2003, suggesting additional analysis strategies for my work, thus providing additional expertise.

Overview of Sections

The dissertation structure, particularly Sections III through VIII, illustrates how I incorporated Abbott's framework in this work. Section III: Community of Therapists, defines and explains occupational therapy's professional culture and social structure. Abbott (1988) suggests that professional grouping strategies promote internal system change with influences that can change the entire system (p 96). The community of therapists groupings included an "old girls' network" in comparison to an "old boys' network." Other groupings include military occupational therapists, and class structure or occupational therapists' society placement.

Section IV: Community Groupings and Portraits, continues defining internal structural groupings, including those occupational therapists readily accepted into the professional community (insiders) and those who were less accepted (outsiders). Describing three major community groupings: (1) occupational therapy theorists and futurists, (2) political movers and (3) sustainers (old and new guard), particular occupational therapists are introduced to the reader, including Ayres, Rood, Reilly, Mosey, Fidler, and Yerxa. Chapter 5, "Political Movers and Sustainers," continues introducing the reader to community therapists, including Wiemer, Cromwell, Gilfoyle, Crampton, Stattel, Welles, Bing, and Llorens. Employing autobiographical and biographical data gathered from 12 occupational therapists' oral histories, interviews, and print sources, and introducing ten occupational therapists in the community of therapists, provides an explanation about how these people chose career paths that contributed to the professionalization of occupational therapy. Their personal stories and words carry the reader to an occupational therapy of 30–50 years ago, a leap that colors how decisions were made to produce a viable occupational therapy. Placing the community of therapists in a larger context, cultural and gender issues are discussed.

Section VI: The Dilemma of Philosophy and Science, and Section VII: Professionalizing: Occupational Therapy and Social Movements, describe how professionalization occurred through philosophical and scientific knowledge development, and its interplay with American social movements in a larger context. Finally, Section VIII: Occupational Therapy's Past Influences It's Present, provides an overview and summary that answers why historical work is as significant to today's occupational therapy as is its science-base. Section VIII informs the reader about what lessons the past holds, perhaps unlocking some doors for occupational therapy and other similar women's professions.

SECTION III: COMMUNITY OF THERAPISTS

Community Culture

The community of therapists, who were internally and externally known as occupational therapy scholars and leaders working toward legitimizing their profession, commonly understood the value of occupational therapy. This section describes occupational therapy's overt and covert community culture, and its divisions and commonalities.

What unified the community and motivated therapists to expand occupational therapy beyond the confines of physician domination? Academically capable therapists from wealthier backgrounds had the resources to study medicine or law, or marry into society. Why did they enter a profession with little prestige? Was it related to limited academic opportunities for women or a true romance with occupational therapy? Can we think that this was a community of cultured women responding to an altruistic, if not religious-like passion to help? Community members Crampton and Wiemer, women open about their beliefs in organized religion, talked about answering "a calling" to help others.

Perhaps members of their generation rebelled against marrying into wealth or "society," seeking careers, lesbian companionship, or living alone. For example, New York occupational therapist Florence Stattel, an old guard member from means who never married, recounted her career motivation and brought light to the motivation of others in her generation, stating:

> I was born in 1916; I'm one year older than the profession. The Stattel women never worked; this was unheard of in the family. This was some-thing mother had to convince father about. I was going against everything. Where could I go in terms of a profession? I could go into nursing in the hospitals. You couldn't get into medicine. A veterinarian was out of the question; I loved animals. I didn't know if social work was what I wanted, because there I wasn't solving problems with my hands.
>
> I said to mother I wish I could find something where I could use my hands and also be helping people. So when I saw the industrial shops and the weaving, and the other things [sic]. They used boxwood to do their carving, and they did chip carving. People came from European backgrounds, they brought with them the skills. (Stattel/Peters oral history, November 20, 1997, lines 140–149; 112–114; 123)

Stattel, like other women in her generation sought an occupation using her hands (therapeutic activities), heart (empathy), and mind (science). Occupational therapy differed from other traditionally female health profes-sions like social work that did not combine these three elements. They fervently believed in what occupational therapy stood for and presented that to society. This conviction was at the heart of the community. The therapists I interviewed represented a portion of those in the larger community. Wiemer believed that the unifying community characteristic was:

> A deep belief in OT, and a strong belief in its truth, and public need for it. All of them [believed that] in their way and in different ways. I think there couldn't be two people more different than Fidler and Crampy [Marion Crampton], for example. But basically, underneath their personalities was this common thread, almost dedication to the betterment of the pro-fession. (Wiemer/Peters oral history, March 18–19, 2003, lines 423–450)

I argue occupational therapists developed into a community to gain professional jurisdiction in the system of professions. The community of therapists is characterized as a group where people had different personal-ities, styles, and venues promoting occupational therapy. These therapists created an implied hierarchy in which few made it to the inner community circle. Cromwell described them as powerful women, stating:

> They were a loaded deck of powerful women. In AOTA they were power-ful women if they chose to be in the mix of decision making, and making

themselves active, regardless of where they lived. You see in a woman's profession everybody has the opportunity for power if they do the work and get in the trenches, because it was women against women. (Cromwell/Peters oral history, April 28–29, 2003, lines 5,664–5,694)

Therapists fell either inside or outside the community of therapists' innermost or core group. Vying for position, either through their own actions or because of group encouragement, the innermost group remained politically visible; they dominated AOTA leadership positions. Colman (1992, 1984) studied some of these decision makers, occupational therapy education program chairs working at the top of their game in the 1950s and 1960s. She identified them as an elite ruling class who differed from the larger membership proletariat. Community members knew each other professionally and socially, often forming extended families. These practices gave select therapists entrance to the community's inner circle. Whether inside or outside the innermost group, the profession's scholars and leaders sought to improve occupational therapy. Elizabeth Yerxa best summarized the occupational therapy community by saying:

There's a very strong sense of community and there's a sense of commitment. I cannot imagine any profession where people all over the world have the degree of commitment that we have. It's a belief, a belief in their profession and the willingness to put themselves out there and really fight for it, because they believe in it so deeply. (Yerxa/Peters oral history, April 21–22, 2003, lines 4,560–4,567)

Old Girls' Network—Professional Women

Professional women coming into their own, the community of therapists used strategies like networking and mentoring to achieve their goals. Brunyate–Wiemer reflects "If you look at this list that you are interviewing, at people, not just OTs, they are very interesting, strong women. And that always intrigues me about OT" (Peters/Wiemer oral history, Mar 18–19, 2003, lines 428–431).

These traditionally female strategies where women sponsor other women, and creating networks out of women's clubs, and sorority practices, and early 20th century suffragists activities where women's networking promoted political change (Rosenow, 1982; Soloman, 1985; Turk, 2004). Community member Stattel describes early occupational therapy influences by saying:

Becky Holdeman who is out in California, she taught at the University of Southern California.[9] She wrote a few books on nursing home care. She worked for the health department. Her mother pushed her baby carriage in the suffrage movement. Many of those women who came out were part of the movement. I felt that it [occupational therapy] came in a time that women's suffrage was also coming out. (Stattel/Peters oral history, November 20–21, 1997, lines 150–155)

Working together professionally, these women found career identities outside their home and family roles. Professional women worked harmoniously or sometimes in competition with each other. Similar to the environments in female sororities and clubs, occupational therapists entered a sisterhood which was characterized as an "old-girls" rather than an "old-boys" network (Colman, 1984; Degler, 1980). Some therapists who excelled in female generated systems learned from their experiences in sorority or club membership and applied this knowledge to occupational therapy. Gilfoyle remembered her late 1950s occupational therapy student internship in Colorado, stating:

> I was a student, so I joined the Colorado OT association. It was small because there weren't many OTs around. It became like an extended family; we all knew each other; we worked together. We would boost our profession together through the association. We all had a common goal, and we'd do things for the common goal. We'd do things for the common good of OT in the state. And it was just a cohesive group, lots of connections because it was small." (Gilfoyle/Peters oral history, Feb 10–11, 2003, lines 166–174)

The community of therapists, a sisterhood of professional women, navigated organizational routines that evolved into an old-girls' network. A system came to exist where women mentored women and men, knowing each other's strengths. Therapists developed each other's leadership and/or scholarly abilities, pushing occupational therapy forward. Using these strategies, occupational therapy began to gain jurisdiction and viability in a larger system of professions. In this connected system, community insiders watched over each other's tutees who had "the right" occupational therapy pedigree.

Senior group members invited younger therapists into the community. Welcoming each other's protégées, senior community members and newcomers supported each other's careers. Many of the members knew each other well, having met at occupational therapy school, often at The Boston School of Occupational Therapy, affiliated at the time with Tufts College, or the Philadelphia School of Occupational Therapy, affiliated with the University of Pennsylvania. Protégés were graduated from these programs and members of the old guard chaired occupational therapy programs like those at the University of Illinois, Chicago; Columbia University; Milwaukee–Downer College; Richmond Professional Institute of the College of William and Mary; New York University; University of Southern California; Washington University School of Medicine; and Wayne State University. As evaluated by this select community, the Boston School of Occupational Therapy (BSOT) was at the top of the old guard list.

East, Midwest and West Coast therapists traveled, renewing relationships at annual conferences and mid-year meetings, by holding key AOTA or AOTF volunteer positions. Working together, often on weekends and evenings, this community greased the engines that ran the profession.

Ruth Brunyate Wiemer remembered AOTA meetings, relaying:

> In thinking about my early indoctrination to AOTA and my privilege of sitting in on the early council on education...at that time it was Bea Wade, Henry [Henrietta Mc Nary], Helen [Willard], and Liz Messick. In those days that council talked about the roots of what should be in our education. They were really talking about fundamentals of OT. They were an interesting group, the committee was small, they all knew each other and they grew up, and shared their agonies together.
>
> And then coming on to the board of management, there again, dialogue was very important. There were only 12 of us there sitting around the table with June Sokolov, Stattel and Fidler, Reilly, and West. There were good dialogues about the profession, not just nitty gritty things, more serious discussions. We had an agenda yes, but the dialogue, the expressions of points of view flowed so freely. They were fascinating meetings really. Yes, it was a precursor of the time when we did a total reorganization and went to the representative assembly, and all that. It was a "we/they" thing. A lot of membership thought the board was too controlling, and what not, and they wanted a more open kind of thing. But to me, much of the value of the other system was the spontaneous dialogues that you lose when you have a more formal...We lost a lot when we lost the spontaneity of sharing. (Brunyate Wiemer/Peters oral history, March 18–19, 2003, lines 5,801–5,827; 43–70)

The closely woven old girls' network illustrates how the community of therapists achieved their goals, promoting the profession politically to physicians and other change agents. Female networking, characteristically different from similar male groups outside of occupational therapy, laid a foundation where women made the decisions, created hierarchies, and dominated leadership. Occupational therapy scholars, who often worked outside the networking box, benefited from insiders' actions because the more verbal leaders found the funding dollars that underwrote scholarly pursuits or kept academic programs alive.

Old Boys' Network—A Minority Group

Occupational therapy's long-standing old girls' network left little room for men. Few men made it into the community's innermost circle. Men gained community introductions based on their occupational therapy educational pedigree, female mentors, or military channels. Having a minority vantage point, these men earned community entrance by displaying their talent, work ethic, and intelligence. Disadvantaged in a close-knit female system, male occupational therapy scholars and leaders seemed peripheral to the inner core. When men did achieve professional authority positions, female committee chairs scrutinized their performances on AOTA and AOTF committees. Wiemer remembered an AOTA board meeting she attended in the 1960s, stating:

> Membership [AOTA] was predominantly female. Among the officers and leadership there was [sic] perhaps 3 or 4 men, and that was all. Dwyer Dundon, Dean Tyndall, Esteban from Puerto Rico, I've forgotten his full name, but he was one of the quiet fellows who all of a sudden came up with a very solid solution to a problem. We had a person to be Marge Fish's[10] replacement, and he wouldn't leave Hawaii. He and Gail were what we would call an item; they were wonderful. (Weimer/Peters oral history, March 18–19, 2003, lines 4,771–4,790)

Immediately following Wiemer, AOTA Presidential candidate Cromwell spoke about her second campaign in the early 1970s, saying:

> I ran against a man the second time when I went for the presidency: Larry Peake. He was military; he was a reservist I think. The vice presidents, two different vice presidents while I was president were fellows, Dean Tyndall from Kalamazoo and Clyde Butz from upstate New York. Weak reeds, I mean they weren't strong board members because they never took a stand, never had a strong position. Nice guys, but just not really leadership types." (Cromwell/Peters oral history, April 28–29, 2003, lines 5,779–5,799)

Robert K. Bing's male perspective about his peers gives a different view, and a look at male relationships while he was preparing to run for his AOTA presidency. Bing states:

> My next fence mending was with Larry Peake. He had tried several times to become president, first time running against Florence Cromwell. She pulled a fast one on him, and he never forgave her. He had gathered a group of OTs together in the early 70s to work up a campaign plan but within a few years it fizzled. The people were not particularly in his camp, just a bunch of dissidents who were unhappy with nearly everyone else.
>
> Phil Shannon had tried to become president, running against Mae Hightower–Van Damm. Phil was in the service at the time and he goofed by not getting official permission from his army superior. When they found out he was a candidate, they told him that if he won he would have to resign. If he lost, it would be recorded on his record. He lost.

With this kind of male record, I really did not think I had much of a chance. It was smack dab in the middle of the feminist movement. But I really think I sneaked by because I did not align myself with any particular faction or group. I sought out Larry Peake at the Philadelphia conference and backed him up against the balcony railing and told him that I fully recognized that I was walking around in a pair of shoes that he very much wanted to wear. I knew that we were only acquaintances, not friends, and I had no intention of appointing him to any committee chair. "I only ask that you wish me well." He looked around and said without emotion, "I can do that." I did receive snide comments from him throughout my tenure but I pretty much ignored them. (Bing/Peters oral history, March 7, 2003, line 1,163–1,186)

Some male occupational therapists formed an annual "mens'group" meeting at AOTA's national conferences in the late 1950s. This developed because the Men's Committee of the New York Occupational Therapy Association requested the formation of an AOTA Men's Committee. When brought to AOTA's March 1949 Board of Management meeting under President Kahmann, the board opposed the request stating: "the profession needed the combined efforts of all occupational therapists working together rather than divided, and that all had the same opportunity and obligation to contribute on both local and national levels. The Board opposed the formation of a men's group as such and urged their cooperative participation in professional activities with women," (Meeting of House of Delegates AOTA, Detroit, August 21, 22, 25, 1949; Board of Management Minutes, New Business, Edna Faeser, Speaker of the House of Delegates, p. 132). Clearly, women leaders took the position that the majority rules. The one compensation the men did get from that meeting was that AOTA would "refrain from referring to OTs as she and her."

After continued efforts, the group formed and eventually dissolved in the 1970s because they were unsuccessful as a support group. Female leaders attended and attempted to set the agenda for this annual meeting. According to female leader Fidler, the organization was unproductive and more social rather than task-oriented. In her opinion the women created a more effective networking system. Bing shared his perspective about the group and Fidler's influence, stating:

There was another form of diverseness that bothered me, male versus female and those who were in and those who were out. By that I mean those who were pro current AOTA administration and those anti current administration. At annual conferences there were all kinds of secret meetings in peoples' hotel rooms, griping about something, fussing about what the president had said or what the Delegate Assembly had recommended. The few men who attended liked to get together and bitch about being in the minority. They had a den mother for several years, Gail Fidler.

She would join them, they would toss her in a blanket, to see if they could hit the ceiling without hurting her. And she would expound for hours about how to take over. In 1973 there was a near coup at the annual conference, but the president got wind of it and put the problem to rest. (Bing oral history, February 11, 2003, lines 190–205)

Gail Fidler, recounting her views about her 1960s occupational therapy male peers, stated:

I think they [male therapists] had more substance than today. I think back and I know some, they're the ones who created the "Men's Group." Well, Manny Brown, and Dwyer Dundon. There seemed to be a lot of pressure amongst guys to have a men's group, because there were so many damn females. They needed a place to just be men together, so they organized the Men's Group. And they kept me informed because I had relationships with each of these guys, and they would talk about their Men's Group.

And I would every once and awhile make a joke about, well you know at least one woman ought to be part of that. So they would meet.

That was the first year that I sat on the Board [AOTA]with Helen Willard.[11] And I wanted to be proper, as proper as I could possibly be; she was quite a woman. Then there was a knock on the door, and they passed a note to Helen Willard. And she looked down the table at me and said, you're wanted outside, so I went outside and closed the door. There was Manny Brown with a cigar; we are about to initiate you into the Men's Group, come with me. I just left the Board meeting, went down and was initiated.

I had to take two drags on that cigar, and was initiated, then went back to the Board meeting, and sat down very proper. So I was involved in the Men's Group all along. They met at conference every year, drank beer and booze. It was a social gathering; I don't think they did anything political. It was a social gathering. (Fidler/Peters oral history, March 6–7, 2003, lines 1,646–1,649; 1,663–1,666; 1,713–1,769)

Community member Llorens also remembers the Men's Group in the 1970s, and its existence parallel in time to the new AOTA Black Caucus group, a different minority group. Llorens, contrasting Fidler's early group memories, reflected that the Men's Group discussed issues rather than held a social gathering meeting from what she understood. Llorens stated:

Dick McCauley was instrumental in trying to get a men's caucus. Many of the men felt disenfranchised, and that they had issues that they wanted to talk about. Well Dick and I talked about that, and about the organization of it. I thought that it was a good idea, I just thought that not enough of the men had issues. I think the main issue was there were so few of them, and some people felt disenfranchised because they were not in the majority, and that was very hard for some. That's hard for a lot of men.

The men in the field tended to do rather well because there were so few of them. So many of the women at the rank and file level were not interested in administration or leadership, and would permit the men, if you will, to do whatever they chose to do in terms of administration and supervision. (Llorens/Peters oral history, April 25–26, 2003, lines 5,198–5,235)

Although touted as apolitical, their gatherings made a political statement and made their presence known to old guard "grand dames." The female community of therapists eventually infiltrated the Men's Group, perhaps changing its original intent. Whether one interprets this as female therapists maintaining a competitive authority (Haskell, 1984; Larson, 1984) or as women protesting larger society issues about male dominance (Degler, 1980; Faludi, 1991; Morantz–Sanchez, 1997), these female therapists were well established, holding senior and junior community positions.

Men's motivations for entering occupational therapy became an issue among female leaders. That turned into a double-edged sword. Savvy occupational therapy leaders knew that expanding and diversifying the profession at the time of the more liberal 1960s and their new societal mindset meant more minority and male recruitment. Yerxa recounted that period in occupational therapy history, stating:

I knew there was a concern nationally that arose from time to time about the lack of men in the field. Efforts were made to try to bring more men into the field, and the percentages stayed pretty constant, even with all the efforts that were made. I think that I was ambivalent about it actually. I think sometimes that people advanced in our field because they were male. They could go right to the top without having the struggles that some women did in order to make their way, and I think that was unfair. But otherwise I think it's a puzzle to me about why we haven't been able to attract more men to the field, and why it remained constant in spite of all these efforts that we've made.

And in some respects, I think, I believe that maybe what we do is very aligned with being a woman. Which to me is a much more female cultural fit, and not a good fit with traditional male roles. (Yerxa/Peters oral history, April 21–22, 2003, lines 2,009–2,056)

Because they didn't represent as much of the minority, male occupational therapists often chose the male dominated military that led to advancement or career opportunities. It also proved a vehicle for female therapists to achieve and hold top positions.

Military Occupational Therapists

Occupational therapy women, and men trained or worked in the military, formed another community grouping. The military proved a particularly good training ground for women, eliminating some civilian gender barriers like promotion opportunities. Male military therapists gained advanced educational opportunities and ultimately reported to the community insiders. Military occupational therapists entered the community of therapists and diversified its class structure. Rather than old money giving one inner circle entrance, high military ranking provided an alternate entrance to the coveted community. Senior military women officers learned that their rank meant authority and brought this to the profession. Women like Winifred Kahmann, Ruth Robinson, and Wilma West, holding senior ranking military positions in World War II, later became AOTA presidents. Community members Cromwell and Welles recalled this community of therapists in the following dialogue:

> Cromwell: Well, some of our leaders were the leaders of the military. Ruth Robinson was the head of the Corps, wasn't she Carlotta?
>
> Welles: Yes
>
> Cromwell: And Willie [West] had been in, and Mary Reilly had been in. Reilly, well she was still a reservist, after 20 years she retired as a major. Well you see the military was a good decision for a man coming through an OT program. To go into the military and get paid for it, their education. And then they were rotated in [sic] all the various bases. And those OT programs in the military were good. Carl Sundstrom, Phil Shannon [sic]. And you see, we got many of those guys though our graduate program [University of Southern California]. Mary [Reilly] made a deal, [and] somehow or other with the SCO [Senior Commanding Officer] to have the guys, to have OTs get more education you see.
>
> Myra McDaniel stayed in her whole career in the military [sic] and was at various bases. And Skip [Maryelle] Dodds, you know there were a lot of people that were officers of AOTA, so that they were active in the profession. They were active in the development of programs, they had their staff all go to get master's degrees. You know, that sort of thing.
>
> Corky [Cordelia] Meyers was military. Yes, and then she came to us and was the editor of AJOT.[12] Myra McDaniel was treasurer. Willie [Wilma West] was still in the picture.
>
> Welles: She was at Walter Reed.
>
> Cromwell: They didn't have OT in the Army before. There were no OTs in the military until Winnie Kahmann started the War Emergency Course.
>
> Welles: But from World War I, there were always a few. They didn't really maneuver anything, but there have always been a few military.

Cromwell: They were reconstruction aides, but that was eons ago.
  Welles: That was eons ago, yes, but they were OTs.
Cromwell: But the war was the impetus.
  Welles: Winnie was, Winnie Kahmann was the one who got the whole thing going. (Cromwell and Welles/Peters oral history, April 28–29, 2003, lines 5,508–5,660 and 5,251–5,276)

In this environment, therapists gained skills in a male-dominated system. Female officers learned that ranking broke gender barriers that civilian occupational therapists faced. Old girls' network rules worked well in the military and they were later applied to the profession. One example is Kahmann's AOTA presidency from 1947 to 1952, which broke the long-standing tradition of male physicians holding that office. Prepared by government service, former military trained therapists held federal and state health care administrative positions. For example, West was influential in her job at the Maternal and Child Health Bureau, and supported occupational therapy with research dollars. This in turn worked well for former military co-worker Reilly, who, like West, served under Kahmann. Reilly, while pursuing an academic career, put the Bureau's money to good use. Fidler, serving in a civilian military position during the war years, also worked closely with West, and used government dollars to promote groundbreaking, theoretically–oriented, continuing education workshops in mental health occupational therapy. These leaders, through their long-standing interconnections, forged a new occupational therapy.

Society Placement

Community insiders believed that upper class and upper-middle class social placement added to community sovereignty and occupational therapy's visibility. For example, traditionally, and still in the 1950s, occupational therapy academic program directors recruited "well bred" educated women like themselves, holding degrees from top private women's colleges. This somewhat biased action perpetuated the idea that proper young, white-gloved, Anglo Saxon women from upper-middle class roots understood that serving society overrode any real need for financial remuneration. These women came to occupational therapy to help rather than to pursue monetary success. Wiemer stated:

Most of the early OTs had some kind of income behind them. I didn't, my era was depression graduate. But before us, the Susie Slagle's of the world had some resources.[13] Clare Spackman was a very rich gal; my understanding was she was. One funny story about Clare. She had a beautiful big portrait of a young boy; it was an antique by a famous painter. It didn't fit [the space], so she cut it off. (Wiemer/Peters oral history, March 18–19, 2003, lines 498–509)

Community member Stattel spoke about others, stating:

Eleanor Clarke Slagle was influential. There was Marjory Taylor that [sic] started the Milwaukee–Downer school. There was Helen Willard, and before her Mrs. Robeson. Helen [Willard] had just come in when I was entering [the Philadelphia School] in 1936. She was a graduate of Mount Holyoke as Willie [West] was a graduate. So those girls had a level above. Bea [Wade] came from Iowa. Henrietta [Mc Nary] came from Milwaukee, her father was a doctor in the Spanish American War, a delightful gentleman, and so she came from background. Sue Barnes came from a medical family. The St. Louis school was started with a strong medical influence, the Barnes Building at Washington University. Charlotte Bone was the first editor of AJOT and her father was a prominent physician in Boston. She was in the Providence art group doing fine jewelry work. She ended up in occupational therapy. Mrs. Greene was a prominent social leader in Boston, and she headed the school.[14] Boston was always in competition with Philadelphia. They were the same social groups of women who were starting those groups. (Stattel/Peters oral history, November 20–21, 1997, lines 57–59; 310– 324)

Occupational therapy class, ethnicity, and racial diversity started changing, although slowly in the 1950s, and increasingly in the 1960s through the 1970s. The GI educational funding continued diversifying enrollment that previously brought more men into the profession when they returned from World War II a decade earlier. The 1960s feminist movement also increased awareness that women's careers outside the home meant increased autonomy. Although class structure changed, old money roots ran deep in the leadership of occupational therapy.

Crampton, Stattel, Wells, and Wiemer spoke about their socioeconomic roots, implying, but never fully stated, their financial and educational resources. They did, however, speak about summer homes, house staff, extensive travel, professional parents helping those less fortunate, and formal coming-out parties. Community member Stattel entered occupational therapy school after briefly doing secretarial work. She talked about her class heritage growing up on Long Island, New York, describing her family's "country" farm or estate. Stattel described her Alsace–Lorraine immigrant family origins as differing slightly from the original wealthier caste of Anglo-Saxon settlers. Such backgrounds determined social prestige and acceptance in early 20th century New York, stating:

The Kings Park community, my parents lived out there in about 1906. I was born in a large 16-room farmhouse that my grandfather bought. It was made into a farm of 82 acres. Now that farm became half of the village of Kings Park, and the railroad station. The town had a caste system too, and we were the second caste. The Smiths, they were the early

English settlers, were the first caste. We were the early German–French accommodation, European settlers in the 1820s. My great-grandfather came over 79 years before the Civil War; the union was very new then. I never thought about this until the [Kings Park, New York] museum asked me to come back and do the family history." (Stattel/Peters oral history, November 20–21, 1997, lines 85–88; 171–181)

Because they were depression-era babies, other community members remembered family for tunes lost or never seen. Those seeking funds resourcefully found their tuition dollars for their occupational therapy education. For example, Yerxa earned academic scholarships to fine private universities. Bing and Cromwell used the GI Bill for their advanced education. Others, like Fidler and Gilfoyle, worked their way through school. Families also played an important role. The Llorens family, an African-American family with limited economic resources, stressed the importance of college educations to Lela and her sister, who both earned graduate degrees.

Resourceful middle and lower-middle class therapists captured academic scholarships while working their way through school, or using military educational benefits. Commonly, their families believed that their children needed a college education. They were progressive for their times, considering that the majority of 1940s and 1950s young women did not have college degrees. Conventionally, family resources went to the male child's education who was then expected to provide for his future family. Once educated, young therapists faced other hurdles to their community entrance.

A predominantly white, middle and upper-middle class group of women, the community accepted racial and cultural diversity on an individual basis based on intelligence or a "right" fit. Academic program directors, powerful women and community members, often introduced the most gifted students to their circle. Rarely publicly stated, if at all, little room existed for men or women of color in this primarily female community of educated white women therapists. Ironically, this practice echoed class bias, because old-money occupational therapists supported liberal humanitarian or good works for the disenfranchised, but secretly coded who they would accept into their professional ranks.

Occupational therapy's founding Anglo-Saxon old-money myth lingered into the 1950s, creating a general tone which reflected control by a wealthier class system. This tone slowly changed in the 1960s, and ethnic diversity slowly crept into the professional fold.

Breaking cultural barriers, white Jews had easier entrance than Blacks to the circle, based on actions of sponsors who brought new people into the community. Even non-Jewish community members were mistaken for being Jewish because of their assertiveness or other negative stereotypes. Community member Gail Fidler, described her ethnic background as "a mixture of everything, German, English; not Jewish, everybody thinks I am." (Fidler/Peters oral history, March 6–7, 3003, lines 3,031–3,033)

Fidler, recalled her consultant position at Springfield State Hospital in Maryland, telling the following vignette:

> Springfield, yes, had a wonderful, wonderful superintendent. Every Christmas the staff put on a Christmas play for patients. I said that's ass backwards. It is the patients who should put on the Christmas pageant for the staff. So I advocated and advocated, and the staff got furious with me. And they complained about this New York Jew who came down to get rid of Christianity. (Fidler/Peters oral history March 6–7, 2003, lines 3,064; 3,058–3,070)

Lower-middle class and poorer students entered occupational therapy academic programs via academic scholarships to private universities or less costly education in the state college/university systems. Occupational therapy slowly diversified, fueled by women giving other women opportunities. Community insiders like Willard, Wade, Spear, and Fish, all academic program directors, mentored newer arrivals into community ways and "proper" behavior. Wiemer remembered her mentors Willard and Spackman when she said:

> I think one of the things I learned from them was yes, you immerse your-self in your profession, in a sense you marry it, you give your all to it. But you have to live another life as well, and you have to build a comfortable lifestyle. Unless it's enriched somehow, you won't be a very good therapist. They knew how to pack it off for the summer, go up to the lake and live their life. They knew how to go off to Europe and have fun. (Wiemer/ Peters oral history, March 18–19, 2003, lines 482–492)

Carlotta Welles, a Willard and Spackman peer, added other insights, recalling their year working together at the Philadelphia School. Capturing Spackman's community placementwas secondary to Willard's status, Welles explained:

> Oh, Helen [Willard] and Clare [Spackman], well Helen was kind of a queen. I worked for them for a year. You had to figure out what Helen wanted and do it Helen's way, but she was very gracious and not pers-nickety. She wasn't the queen bee in the sense of being lordly to every-body. We all went along with what she said and wanted; it was a pleasant year. I was fonder of her than I was of Clare. Clare was organized, gra-cious, and factual; she wasn't warm and not so interesting; she was alright. (Welles/Peters oral history, April 28–29, 2003, lines 3384–3412)

Beatrice Wade, a community insider along with Helen Willard, was another well-placed therapist. Gillete, a former student of hers, remembered:

She was a truly remarkable woman, everyone who knew her would tell you, unless they were scared of her. She herself came from two families who were the earliest settlers in Iowa. The town of Dorothy, Iowa, is named for her maternal grandfather. Her family was intimately involved in the politics, the education and mental health system of Iowa. They were mostly lawyers, and her father eventually became the administrator for the mental health system of Iowa. She grew up assuming the life of public service, an avid John Kennedy Democrat. She had a style in social life that meant she was listened to. (Peters/Gillette oral history, January 29, 2003, lines 98–132)

Wade, Willard, and Spackman exemplified old-money roots, and set the old-guard community view and standards for proper young women entering occupational therapy. For change to occur, however, the community diversified and expanded.

In this section I introduced and explored the community of therapists' culture, beliefs, and functions. Culturally, the community of therapists was a group of professionally educated women forming old girl networks. The community divided, based on insider and outsider status, and their roles as occupational therapy scholars or leaders. Community insiders and occupational therapy leaders like Wade and West created opportunities for younger therapists and used their own political connections to promote the profession. Community outsiders like Ayres and Reilly—those not supporting AOTA policy lines—often channeled their energy into scholarly activities like expanding the body of knowledge. Male occupational therapists like Bing represented an occupational therapy minority group. Occupational therapists' social placement, primarily as white, middle-class women, often derived from old-money roots. Class and racial diversity grew, initially within a military environment, or later by responding to a changing society, particularly in the 1960s through 1970s. Understanding the community as a whole, their goal was to create a viable occupational therapy profession.

In the next section, I further define community groupings, introducing the reader to specific occupational therapy theorists, and political movers and sustainers. I also show how their beliefs and actions moved the profession to become a science-based profession.

SECTION IV: COMMUNITY GROUPINGS AND PORTRAITS

Theorists and Futurists

Occupational therapy theorists are the scholars who developed a theoretical or rationale-based body of knowledge. Believing a balance between philosophy and science possible, theoretically-minded therapists introduced their work to mixed response and limited funding sources. Why did these scholars stand outside the inner most community circles, considering they, like community insiders, worked toward making occupational therapy a bona fide profession? Does their exclusion support the thesis that expanding a knowledge base was too narrow of a focus to professionalize occupational therapy? If so, what purpose did outsiders serve to the community?

Theorists broke a long tradition of physician-authored occupational therapy literature and thus are historically significant. Through their writings, they challenged not only the medical establishment politically, but also questioned whether that body of knowledge fit occupational therapy. Theorists argued for an intellectually separate occupational therapy that had a broader knowledge base. No longer medicine's "handmaid," the profession's theorists developed new occupational therapy frames of reference like occupational behavior, the developmental approach, and sensory integration.

Although old-guard traditionalists like Willard and Wade fought physiatrists in the late 1940s into the 1950s, they probably didn't see occupational therapy theoretical knowledge as separate from medicine's. Physicians like neurologist Adolf Meyer (1922) laid occupational therapy's philosophical foundation, linking moral treatment and life rhythms. Old-guard members supported these principles, arguably excluding the "colder" 1950s' and 1960s' interest in objective science. Secondly, baccalaureate-level, old-guard therapists may have felt unequipped to understand or execute scientific research. We are left to speculate because many of these traditionalists are no longer available to interview.

Deciding on dollar distribution, community insiders searched for a philosophic rather than a scientific core in the 1970s, culminating in AOTA's funding a controversial philosophical-base project that lasted through three presidencies consisting of Jerry Johnson, Mae Hightower Van Damm, and Robert K. Bing's in the 1980s. I will discuss what Bing described as occupational therapy's historical "mistake" in the next section. There is no parallel project addressing occupational therapy's scientific base.

Swimming upstream, theorists and futurists continued asking thought-provoking questions, challenging an outdated occupational therapy, still in medicine's shadow, in an effort to develop an authentic and autonomous profession. Shifting paradigms, traditional occupational therapy "how to" or "cookbook" approaches listing diagnoses and appropriate craft activities, no longer adequately met scholarly standards. In practice, insider community members did not welcome discourse or changing traditions. Interestingly Wiemer disputed this, stating "Nobody seemed uncomfortable about the dialogues over where we should be. They (occupational therapy leaders) were fundamentally grounded in the concept of OT" (Wiemer/Peters oral history, March 18–19, 2003, lines 438–441). However, when Wiemer discussed the concept of occupational therapy, she spoke about a philosophical rather than a scientific base, as did other community insiders. The community outsiders challenged the status quo.

Respected and honored for their knowledge contributions, they received AOTA's Slagle lectureships, requiring nomination, support, and inner-community sanction. This was not an easy task, considering some theorists stood outside of the community's innermost circles. Rather than joining inner-community circles, outside theorists functioned individually, limiting those with whom they shared their evolving work. Insider community members saw these theorists as mavericks or rebels, accepting that every family has their "black sheep." Quoted here, Llorens questioned how effective non-conforming strategies for occupational therapy theorists are in the end by saying "Now there have been people who made waves, and didn't stay in the box at all, and yet they haven't been effective in the way they tried to get their message across" (Llorens/Peters oral history, April 25–26, 2003, lines 5,720–5,724).

Candid and outspoken community member Fidler saw this division related to therapists' self-esteem, stating:

> Yes, because we feel so inadequate, one of the things that has bugged me forever is our lack of collegiality, our lack of sharing. We don't share; we don't talk to one another, except in a very closed way at home. And we are very guarded about what we think, and what we're theorizing about. (Fidler/Peters oral history March 6–7, 2003, lines 5,488–5,492; 5,496–5,498)

Elizabeth Yerxa identified other community dividers, including anti-intellectualism and geographic location. Yerxa, a Californian educated in Los Angeles and Boston, stated that initially she felt separate from the East Coast occupational therapy think tank and said "I remember feeling like an outsider because of that (geography) in the beginning. There was definitely a feeling that the people on the East Coast were the establishment and that their ideas tended to dominate" (Yerxa/Peters oral history April 21–22, 2003, lines 3,307–3,314).

Dominant insider occupational therapy leaders did not readily speak about community outsiders. Theorists like A. Jean Ayres, Mary Reilly, and Anne Cronin Mosey were nonconformists. Ayres, Reilly, and Mosey promoted an occupational therapy thinking shift, questioning a long-standing, physician-introduced medical pathology model. Each therapist argued that patients are more than their disease process, which they saw as a reductionistic viewpoint. Innovatively, they spoke about studying normal schoolchildren prior to understanding neurological concerns (Ayres), examining occupational behaviors (Reilly), and learning about theory development (Mosey). Entering new territories, particularly in the 1970s, these therapists and others like Fidler, Llorens, and Gilfoyle developed theoretical rationales for treatment. These women challenged all therapists to think about why they did what they did, going beyond how they specifically treated patients.

Most notably, occupational therapy literature changed. Early 1950s therapist-authored articles spoke about craft techniques and chronicled patient diagnoses. Bing spoke about Willard and Spackman's prominent 1950s textbook, *Occupational Therapy*, and said:

> Look at the first edition of Willard and Spackman, that was put together by authors who were most prominent in the field at the time. Willard and Spackman drew that group together and they pretty well outlined what each one would contribute. Spackman got carried away and made a "cookbook" out of her chapter, thereby infuriating all the others who agreed to write. But that was Spackman, the very epitome of the nit-picking, tweezers crowd. (Bing/Peters oral history, February 6, 2003, lines 96–102)

Inexperienced authors wrote research articles, descriptive in nature, showing first attempts. Some of these authors were limited in their bachelors level education. As more therapists earned graduate degrees, therapist-authored articles changed in content and nature.[15] Doctorally educated occupational therapy authors like Ayres, Mosey, and Reilly wrote about conceptual foundations or rigorous scientific methodologies. Yerxa described these theorists and said:

> Oh, Mary Reilly, oh gosh, yes, I mean she's a boat rocker, well Mosey too, Anne Mosey. I think in many ways they agreed more than they disagreed in terms of this broad idea of occupational therapy. But I think both of them are very authoritarian people. (Yerxa/Peters oral history, April 21–22, 2003, lines 2,930–2,940)

Yerxa spoke about A. Jean Ayres and Mary Reilly and stated:

> There was a lot of controversy about both of them (Ayres and Reilly), and I'm sure that some of it was founded in this anti-intellectualism we have in our field. Who are they to be saying, to be creating this?
>
> And Jean Ayres, a lot of her controversy came not from OT but from Special Education. They (the special educators) saw her as a tremendous threat. I attended a conference at one time for special educators; the way they were pillorying Jean Ayres, I absolutely was just blown away by it. And of course she was an outsider (to education), and I think she was threatening. I think this is because it addressed some of what they thought was their territory, the whole idea of neurology.
>
> Mary Reilly, I think, was considered more of a threat within the field because she was raising questions about this traditional view of science. (Yerxa/Peters oral history, April 21–22, 2003, lines 4,269–4,293)

Outsider theorists, the most elusive of all the community groupings, left their legacy in their books rather than through first-hand accounts (Ayres, 1963, 1972, 1976, 1979; Mosey, 1968a, 1968b, 1973, 1981, 1985, 1986, 1996; Reilly, 1960, 1962, 1974). Community outsiders, those who challenged occupational therapy's long-standing connection to medicine's pathology model and went against community insiders' traditionalist viewpoints to the point of criticism or exclusion, hold an important place in occupational therapy. Their stories about making contributions, speaking out, and exclusion bring another layer to telling about and understanding the profession's development that can be lost. Outsider stories address the fine lines between public and private lives, particularly in the occupational therapy culture where both are blurred. For example, A. Jean Ayres, now deceased, was portrayed as frail by colleagues Llorens and Yerxa, and took peer criticisms to heart. Mary Reilly disengaged from the profession, retiring in the late 1970s, and guards her privacy to this day. Margaret Rood, former University of Southern California occupational therapy academic chairperson, criticized for her theoretical concepts, worked in her later career as a physical therapist and educator. When community members spoke about the youngest theorist in the group, Anne Cronin Mosey, they portrayed a woman genius, but their comments implied a taboo. Writing about outside theorists fairly means presenting both sides of a picture for historical reconstruction rather than voyeurism or perpetuating unfounded gossip.

Not all theorists were outsiders. There are insider scholars like Elizabeth Yerxa and Gail Fidler willing to give firsthand accounts. Solitary at times, like other scholars, Yerxa fits the isolated thinker profile. Yerxa also views occupational therapy broadly and globally, characterizing her as a futurist thinker. Fidler, a scrappy conversationalist when stimulated, is one of the hardest to classify, claiming she was alone, "out on a limb," and "ahead of her time," (Fidler/Peters oral history, March 6–7, 2003, lines 4,340–4,343) debunking any convention or category. Fidler more comfortably identified herself as a leader rather than scholar, seeing so few occupational therapy scholars, and stated:

> I'm a leader. I don't have the credentials to be a scholar, a reasonable scholar.[16] I don't think people with scholarly intent, goals, or attitude choose OT, they choose medicine, they choose law. I think because we're an underclass, we don't project anything strong in terms of opportunities. There isn't anything there. (Fidler/Peters oral history, March 6–7, 2003, lines 4,066–4,079)

Later in this section you will meet theorists and futurists individually, including and in order, Ayres, Rood, Reilly, Mosey, Yerxa, and Fidler. They represent community outsiders and insiders, and commonly asked the difficult questions, challenging a traditional occupational therapy viewpoint.

Political Movers

Political leaders in occupational therapy, generally community insiders, made people connections. These people chose their battles well, deciding who and what professions to ally with, medicine always taking precedence, for better or worse. This meant knowing and appreciating those supporters who helped, rather than hindered, occupational therapy's advancement.

Politically, occupational therapists gained new footing, making their causes known to lawmakers and politicians, recapturing earlier strategies. For example, founder Eleanor Clarke Slagle's brother, a United States Senator from New York, provided entrances into the Washington, DC political life for his sister. Forming a working alliance with First Lady and uman rights activist Eleanor Roosevelt, Slagle moved occupational therapy's causes forward (Lash, 1971, 1972; Quiroga, 1995; Wiesen Cook, 1992). These political entrees set a template for future Washington, DC, and were connections called upon during the post-World War II years. Political and military alliances remained close. President Dwight D. Eisenhower's Western Union Telegram, sent to Lt. Colonel Ruth A. Robinson, AMSC, and President of the American Occupational Therapy Association, on October 20, 1957, illustrated such connections when he said:

> Please give my greetings to the members of the American Occupational Therapy Association assembled in their 40th annual conference. Your association renders splendid service to the nation's sick and disabled through the healing art of physical and mental restoration. As you seek to increase your effectiveness by teaching the principles of occupational therapy to a wide audience. (Bing collection, private papers, 1957)

President Lyndon B. Johnson, like Eisenhower, sent conference greetings to the American Occupational President Ruth Brunyate on October 28, 1965. Johnson wrote "Our nation is on the threshold of major new advances in the conquest of disability and disease. Occupational therapy is a vital part of this total effort" (Brunyate Wiemer collection, private papers, 1965).

Always monitored, the community watched who knew whom, holding these connections like a prized poker hand. Stattel, remembering another Lyndon Johnson connection the year she taught at Texas Woman's University said:

> This goes back to 1970, when I was in Texas, (occupational therapist) Cornelia Watson knew Lyndon Baines Johnson. They bought cattle from him. Cornelia Watson, I forgot her married name, had gone down to Dallas, Texas, and worked. We were working to get occupational therapy in a national health program if national health had gone in at that time. We had it all lined up; then LBJ didn't run. We had worked for almost a year on that. Lady Bird was very active in Texas Woman's University.
>
> They were just starting the Texas OT Association. I was hoping to organize their finances because at the time they didn't have money

invested properly. Bob Bing was down there at that time, he was getting it incorporated. (Stattel/Peters oral history, November 20–21, 1997, lines 507–519)

On another front, a year later AOTA's executive director and occupational therapist Harriet Tiebel wrote a letter to therapist M. Joy Anderson in Kalamazoo, Michigan on April 2, 1971, asking for a political connection. She said:

> Once again I am writing to you to ask your assistance in our communication with your cousin, Congressman Robert Anderson. We want to ask Mr. Anderson to support a bill to be introduced into the House, by him perhaps, amending the Social Security law to include occupational therapy in outpatient services and as a single service in home health agencies. (AOTF Archives, Washington Consulting Services, 1971, Coll RG4, Bx NR 73, File NR 526)

Tiebel further asked whether Joy Anderson would travel to Washington, DC to visit her Congressman cousin William Robert Anderson, and discuss occupational therapy's interests, suggesting possible dates and travel expenses to be paid for by AOTA. Anderson, then Assistant Professor of Occupational Therapy at Western Michigan University responded on April 8, 1971, saying she would be vacationing in England on the suggested meeting dates, but would be returning home to Tennessee from May 21 through June 20. She further stated:

> However, I have already written to Robert and asked for his assistance again. Health care is a top priority on everyone's list, and I am sure it is very much a concern of Robert's too. I explained to him that you would like to meet with him again, that you had invited me but I could not come, and that you wanted to discuss amending the Social Security law. I feel sure he will be glad to meet with you and others.
>
> I am sorry I will not be able to come to Washington to meet with you and I appreciate the invitation. It would have been good to see Robert, and also to help in any way I could. Please let me know if I can be of any other assistance. (Washington Consulting Service, 1971, Coll RG 4, Bx NR 73, File NR 526)

Anderson concluded her letter with regrets about Tiebel's AOTA resignation. This resignation is another political move linked to insider community decision makers.

Insiders argued about moving AOTA's office from 251 Park Avenue South in a high rent district in New York to Bethesda, Maryland because they thought it would bring occupational therapy closer to the Washington, DC beltway and other health care professions' headquarters. Cromwell considered this successful move one of the more positive achievements of her AOTA presidency. Tiebel did not move with the association. Apparently community insiders decided that she was a poor fit for the more aggressive and increasingly political organization. Former AOTA Secretary and board member Gillette recalls:

> Two things come to mind when I was on the board, the move to Washington, and as part of that we removed the executive director. I don't think we had done that before, but we did ask for a resignation. A lovely woman, we all adored her; she simply didn't have the leadership skills that the organization needed at that time, in the board's assessment. More and more was happening in Washington and we felt we should be a part of, modernistic things. (Gillette/Peters oral history, January 29, 2003, lines 770–785)

Wiemer remembers Tiebel, comparingher to her predecessor Fran Helmig, AOTA executive director in 1964. Weimer stated:

> Fran couldn't continue; Harriet Tiebel was in my presidency. Tiebel was less forceful, Fran was a business woman, quite firmly spoken. I would say Tiebel was more reticent. But we had a terrible time, we couldn't get any executive director. We tried hard looking for one; at that time people didn't want it. (Wiemer/Peters oral history, March 18–19, 2003, lines 2,646–2,658)

Wilma West stood on the community's top rung of the political ladder. She, along with other community leaders, made decisions supporting occupational therapy's place in health care and rehabilitation. In the 1950s, old-guard academic program directors like Beatrice Wade, Helen Willard, Marjorie Greene, Henrietta McNary, Marjorie Fish, and Marion Spear maintained much influence internally. AOTA Director of Education, Virginia Kilburn, a Wellesley graduate, as were other community members like Willard and Crampton, kept the academic political fires stoked at the staff level. Stattel recalled politically capable Mary Merrit, working at the New York State Department of Health in 1939 by saying"Yes, she [Merrit] was very influential along with Eleanor Clarke Slagle. A very early person, and I believe she was one of the reconstruction aides" (Stattel/Peters oral history November 20–21, line 310).

Other 1950s and 1960s leaders, Ruth Robinson, Myra McDaniel, active and reserve military, and Winfred C. Kahmann, held AOTA national volunteer offices, all providing a backing to 1960s and 1970s leaders, Ruth Brunyate Wiemer and Florence Cromwell. Elnora Gilfoyle, a younger-generation community member, came into her political peak in the 1980s. Illustrating mentorship and community circles, Wiemer, a close colleague of West and a Robinson admirer, graduated from the Philadelphia School under the watchful eyes of mentor Helen Willard. To this day, Wiemer refers to her former professor as Miss Willard, reflecting a special place in her heart.

Remembering Willard through photographs, Wiemer's eyes welled up with emotion when sharing a photograph showing a proud Willard standing next to her protégée.She stated:

> This is a precious picture, Helen Willard and me at my Slagle. Yes, she was just so precious. She took me to dinner that night. We always wore evening dresses. Helen was an incredible woman. I think one of the things that has always drawn me to OT is the caliber of persons that your peers are. (Wiemer/Peters oral history, March 18–19, 2003, lines 3,446–3,488; 423–426)

Wiemer and West entered Washington, DC political circles, making their mark in the 1960s: West at the Department of Health, and Wiemer, shrewdly hiring Russell Dean, Director of Washington Consulting Service (WCS) during her AOTA presidential years. According to Wiemer, Dean's lobbying effectively introduced occupational therapy to United States Senators and Congress members in the late 1960s and 1970s. They initiated a political campaign, meeting regularly and brainstorming about occupational therapy's best placement in reference to insurance coverage and manpower needs.

West and Wiemer's Washington, DC successes and perceived failures were one entry point (Wiemer, 1972a, 1972b, 1978; Weimer & West, 1970). Other community members in the 1970s like Gilfoyle, Llorens, and Cromwell broke new ground bringing change to the public school system, and community mental health systems that redefined occupational therapists' roles and workplaces.

Sustainers

Occupational therapy sustainers provided the architectural infrastructure for theorists and political front-liners. Sustainers mediated and moderated occupational therapy's growth wisely. Working well with other professions like medicine, physical therapy, psychology, and social work, they demonstrated occupational therapy's worth. Internally they sustained occupational therapy through their countless volunteer hours and also contributed financially when it was needed.

Characteristically, sustainers fell into two groupings: the insider old-guards and the new minority. Old-guard sustainers like Florence Stattel, Marion Crampton, and Carlotta Welles lived adventurous lives as single women coming from independent yet discreet wealth. They were the anonymous financial donors. Worldly, speaking foreign languages, having received private secondary educations, they traveled the world with their large circle of occupational therapy female friends. These 1930s graduates held degrees from the finest private liberal arts women's universities prior to their occupational therapy education. They used their social connections judiciously.

Knowing influential members of fashionable society like politicians, business executives, physicians, and lawyers, they brought occupational therapy into new drawing rooms. These sustainers worked anonymously and humbly which was advantageous for the little-known profession of occupational therapy. These occupational therapy Grande dames worked behind the scenes.

The minority sustainers, having less affluent backgrounds, supported occupational therapy differently. Lela Llorens broke new ground and old stereotypes when she entered the community of therapists. Llorens' academic talent stood out to Marion Spear, Wayne State University occupational therapy program director. Spears, a Boston School graduate, used her blue-blood academic pedigree to pave the way for Llorens by introducing her to influential therapists like Boston School alumna Wilma West. West, an avid occupational therapy talent scout, supported Llorens' career development and community placement.

Robert K. Bing, a community outsider, broke new ground for white men in occupational therapy. Bing's accomplishment as an occupational therapy historical scholar, culminating in his Eleanor Clarke Slagle lecture, paralleled his political, although controversial, position as AOTA's first and only male occupational therapist president. Community old-guard Beatrice Wade, Bing's undergraduate academic chair at the University of Illinois, assured him community introductions and a career-long sounding board.

In many ways, sustainers were occupational therapy's working backbone. Taking on countless AOTA and AOTF volunteer hours, sustainers worked diligently, maintaining and improving the growing organizations. Whether they promoted occupational therapy in their work environments, or talked about it to a larger and influential public, providing their own money when necessary, they believed in the profession. Common to all other community members, the theorists and political movers as sustainers demonstrated that occupational therapy worked and was vitally necessary to society.

Community Portraits

I will introduce 10 members of the community of therapists, who are occupational therapy's theorists, political movers, and sustainers. Identifying these insider and outsider scholars and leaders and what motivated them to change occupational therapy to a science-based profession provides a clear illustration of how each one influenced the profession. Gail Fidler and Elizabeth Yerxa are two theorists and futurists. Ruth Brunyate, later Brunyate–Wiemer, Florence Cromwell, and Elnora Gilfoyle are the political movers. Sustainers, representing the largest cohort, are old-guard members Marion Crampton, Florence Stattel, and Carlotta Welles; and new-guard members, Lela Llorens and Robert Bing. I will also discuss theorists who these 10 therapists spoke about because of their place in occupational therapy history. Therapists A.

Jean Ayres, Margaret Rood, Anne Mosey, and Mary Reilly broadened the thinking of these scholars' and leaders' thinking and influenced occupational therapy and its trajectory toward the goal of becoming a science-based profession. Although I have created insider and outsider groupings based on data analysis, these categories are subject to interpretation and challenge. For example, some whom I identify as outsiders, like Ayres and Reilly, Gilfoyle identified as insiders in this statement, saying:

> I had a group of friends, but it wasn't the inner circle they used to have. These were the people who were idolized. Well, I think Bob Bing saw himself as one. I think Jean Ayres was, I think Mary Reilly was. I think Ruth Brunyate was; Jerry Johnson was. I think it sort of stopped at Jerry Johnson. I think Betty Yerxa was in some ways. Alice Jantzen in an interesting way. (Gilfoyle/Peters oral history, February 10–11, 2003, lines 3,056–3,067)

Each portrait reflects an introduction to an occupational therapy theorist, political mover, or sustainer. Considering that each person's career spanned 35 or more years, these portraits skim over their full careers and lives. The reader will then understand these leaders' and scholar's differences and commonalities. Some differences included geographic location, age, gender, race, ethnic origins and family background. Of the nine women and one man providing oral histories, an unexpected common personal characteristic was their strong ties to their fathers. Although a few spoke about both parents, all talked about how their fathers mentored their critical thinking abilities. The reader will notice a shift between those therapists who gave first person accounts and those whom I learned about through their writings or others recollections. When writing about people whom I visited, I will include pertinent environmental observations, including cherished artifacts that placed these people in the context of their environment or history. Unifying them is their common belief in occupational therapy and their significant contributions in helping create new emplacements in the system of professions. While establishing occupational therapy in this larger system, these were the scouts who charted new territory.

Outsider Theorists: Ayres, Rood, Reilly, and Mosey

Occupational therapy theorists Ayres, Rood, Reilly, and Mosey were considered some of the profession's brightest and most capable scholars. Paradoxically, either by choice or exclusion, each woman remained outside the community of therapists' innermost circle. They argued the merits of an objective science, a view that challenged the caring philosophical vantage point that community insiders believed. Creating an internal tension, did outsider theorists help or hinder occupational therapy's professional development?

A. Jean Ayres

A. Jean Ayres (1920–1988), a "therapist, scholar, scientist, and teacher" (Bowman, 1989, p. 480), formulated a theoretical basis for the practice then called "sensory integration." Ayres helped children who experienced learning problems similar to those that that she had struggled with as a child in rural south central Visalia, California. Although she developed more than 20 standardized tests and published more than 50 scholarly papers and books, Ayres was excluded from, rather than embraced by, the community of therapists. Why did more recognition come after her death when AOTF created an award in her name?

Well educated, Ayres earned her occupational therapy bachelors (1945) and master's degree (1954) at the University of Southern California (USC). USC was the western occupational therapy think tank that awarded the first master's degree in occupational therapy to Wilma West. Ayres earned her doctor of philosophy degree, when few therapists had master's, in educational psychology (1961) at USC. Was the Ayres controversy related to her theoretical work, perhaps too far afield from known occupational therapy practice, or was it related to her intellectualism? Lela Llorens spoke about some of Ayres' challenges as she remembered them and stated:

> On the West Coast Ayres was getting her doctorate in neurophysiology and she really wasn't all that interested in identifying herself as an occupational therapist. And, for quite a long time, she dropped the OTR [occupational therapist registered] from her credentials. She just went with her PhD. She faced a lot of hostility from the East Coast people for her ideas and to some extent for the way in which they felt she didn't really warm up to anybody. I mean she had her own thinking, she had her own way of doing things and you could sort of take it or leave it.
>
> When Jean Ayres was at what I would call the height of her game in terms of sensory integration, teaching, and trying to teach the rest of the profession, she was greeted with real hostility in one of the sessions. She didn't stop doing it, but she was practically sick, and she was fragile. She met with a lot of hostility from people who didn't want to believe what she was saying. Mary Reilly was one of those people. (Llorens/Peters oral history, April 25–26, 2003, lines 6,309–6,321; 6,723–6,734)

Similar to Llorens' memories, Yerxa reflected:

> I did have contact with Jean Ayres. I don't think she was on faculty when I was there [USC], but I knew her, I knew her when I was a student [at USC]. Jean Ayres, I think of her a lot. She reminds me of Jane Goodall in many respects. They sort of appear to be similar. You can see the similarity, and they had similar personalities, in the sense that I don't think she ever intended to rock the boat, but she did. And I think she was hurt

by a lot of people's reactions because she just wanted to help children very deeply. She wasn't out to make a reputation for herself, as I ever saw it. And I think she did help a lot of children to improve with her work. (Yerxa/Peters oral history, April 21–22, 2003, lines 882–886 and 4,313–4,325)

Gilfoyle spoke about Ayres' disconnection to AOTA, along with another theorist and outsider Josephine Moore. She stated:

When Jean Ayres was at her prime, she was very angry at the Association, and so was Jo Moore. I lost a little respect for them because of the things they used to say about the Association. Jean Ayres didn't feel the association supported her with her research. The association didn't give her enough money support. Willie tried very hard to get her some foundation support. Same with Jo Moore, and it's the squeaky wheel that gets the grease. I don't want to be a squeaky wheel. I looked at them and I thought, that's what they are doing. They're whining. History repeats itself. (Gilfoyle/Peters oral history, Feb. 10–11, 2003, lines 2,384–2,407)

Offering another dimension, Gilfoyle remembered Ayres' work influencing her own pediatric theoretical work and stated:

I got real interested in child development and how children learn to move. Mary Reilly and Jean Ayres were the two who began to write about it. I met Jean when I began to use all her stuff. She has some really early tests out before the sensory integrative battery that we used at the University of Colorado and at Children's Hospital in Denver. She [Ayres] was beginning to work with children with minimal brain dysfunction, and that was all that was going on in the United States at the time. There was a lot of money for research. So people were beginning to finance through the Children's Bureau, through Health and Education, it was HEW at the time, and she was getting money to do her post doc. (Gilfoyle/Peters oral history, February 10–11, 2003, lines 780–789; 795–803; 479–495)

Yerxa compared Reilly and Ayres, identifying an important theoretical convergence, that both wrote about normal human beings. She stated:

Both she [Ayres] and Mary Reilly are very interesting. They are totally divergent. Jean Ayres doesn't have conflicts with anyone, but they had intellectual conflicts. They both were deeply concerned about practice.
    Both of them created a whole conceptual framework, dealing with people, human beings who were normal human beings, not people who had disabilities. Ultimately they wanted it to be applied to people who had problems. They had to back up and define a whole area about human beings that was the foundation for their practice. Jean Ayres' book

on Sensory Integration is not about pathology. It's about human beings and how important sensory integration is to their developmental process.(Yerxa/Peters oral history, April 21–22, 2003, lines 4194–4214)

Although others, like Llorens in child mental health, and Moore in adult rehabilitation, wrote about neurological rehabilitation, Ayres' neurological theories remained controversial. Ayres spent her career concerned about neurologically involved children. Frustrated and performing poorly, these children blended into the school system. Until Ayres identified them, they were undiscovered or underserved by occupational therapists. Llorens, although a colleague, saw herself as an Ayres student. She stated:

I had heard her speak sometime in the 60s when I was at the Lafayette Clinic. Over the years I tried to hear her because it took listening to her, it took reading her books. I felt I was 10 years behind her in terms of understanding what she was talking about. And I would carry her books with me whenever I had to take an airplane trip anyplace because that was a block of time that I could spend to read and understand what she was trying to teach us.(Llorens/Peters oral history, April 25–26, 2003, lines 1,638–1,649)

To leave the reader thinking that Ayres stood outside the community of therapists is misleading. Gilfoyle saw Ayres as a part of the occupational therapy community or family. Although contradictory, all occupational therapists were overtly part of the larger sisterhood, including outsiders. Covertly, outsiders had and knew their community placement. Gilfoyle stated:

Within the OT community you strategize as peers. With OT, even with Jean Ayres, it's more peer strategizing. Everyone has this common belief system, for the common good. We believed in each other, we supported each other. There wasn't a difference in hierarchy in who we were; we were all equal from my perspective. And there was a lot about who we are as people. (Gilfoyle/Peters oral history, February 10–11, 2003, lines 1,807–1,825)

When comfortable, Ayres welcomed connections, both professional and social. Llorens describes Ayres meeting her daughter, Maria, in the 1970s. Llorens, then a faculty member at the University of Florida, Gainesville, invited Ayres to lecture. She recalled:

We had her come to our house for dinner and Maria met her. She was so kind and gentle with Maria. She read her 4th grade paper on the brain. Maria thought it was wonderful too, because she grew up with all these people like Barbara Knickerbocker, Gail Fidler, and Jean Ayres. (Llorens/Peters oral history, April 25–26, 2003, lines 1,627–1,636)

Ultimately above all divisions, Ayres held a place in the community, albeit that of an outsider. Because she was a recognized theorist, peers talked about her scholarship and how she introduced new tradition breaking ideas.

Margaret Rood

Rood's neurophysiological treatment approach examined how activating, facilitating, and inhibiting voluntary or involuntary muscle action occurs through a reflex arc. Using this approach, specific therapeutic exercise patterns and sensory stimulations like vibration, brushing muscles, and joint compression enhance learning a correct response (Huss, 1977). Cromwell compared Rood's and Ayres' work and stated:

> Jean Ayres and Rood had a different kind of way of going at the nervous system. It was unfortunate that they were both at the same time. I think Ayres was more likely to attract [the] OTs because she was working with children primarily. She presented simple neurological principles than stuff that Roody was talking about. The Rood theory was a very special neurological theory. OTs weren't doing as much with the whole body as her theory demanded. The brushing and the pounding, and stuff like that, and some people who worked with stroke patients used them. But she worked a lot with the PTs with lower extremity stuff. (Cromwell/ Peters oral history, April 28–29, 2003, lines 7,557–7,572)

Initially an occupational therapist, Margaret Rood, or Roody to her friends, left occupational therapy for physical therapy. Such a move was not unheard of, but other therapists like Helen Willard and Josephine Moore studied both disciplines and didn't leave. Cromwell shared Rood memories and said:

> She left USC and went to Stanford and took her Certificate/Master's in PT. And then she started getting more and more interested in neurology. And the PTs would have nothing to do with her. After she went to PT school and got her master's at Stanford, she came back to the LA area. And that's when she was doing work with the Crippled Children [organization] out in the desert driving around.(Cromwell/Peters oral history, April 28–29, 2003, lines 923–964; 7,486–7,490)

Yerxa remembered Rood orienting her to the Elks Crippled Children's job and stated:

> After I graduated, my second job was with the Elks, and I was based in Lancaster, California. As part of my orientation, I went down to Palm Springs and went around with Margaret Rood while she was treating all these children. And we drove about 110 miles an hour across the desert while we went to these little shacks where these children were

found, and everything was just fascinating. (Yerxa/Peters oral history, April 21–22, 2003, lines 561–572)

Energetic, with so much to share, did Rood think occupational therapy too limited, or did she leave after receiving the community's cold shoulder because people thought that her theories were too avante gard? As with other outsider theorists, Rood's non-conforming thinking and theoretical work caused occupational therapists not to greet her kindly. Unfortunately, physical therapists also questioned her ideas. Cromwell talked about Rood's exclusion and stated:

The PTs were as much divided on her, what she was about, as the OTs. They just laughed her out of Rancho [a well-known Los Angeles rehabilitation center]. Rancho wouldn't even let her cross the threshold, they, orthopedists and PTs there, and OTs too. They just thought she was kind of a crazy woman, they were just dreadful to her, and she was still functioning [as an occupational therapist].

There are still people here who are ardent Rood specialists, among PT particularly. Roody came back [to the University of Southern California] and was chair of PT the second time and some of those faculty whom I still know, are ardent Rood supporters. (Cromwell/Peters oral history, April 28–29, 2003, lines 7,494–7,538; 7,599–7,600)

Cromwell, doing her master's degree studies, and Yerxa, working on her undergraduate degree, remembered Rood chairing USC's occupational therapy program in the early 1950s prior to Harriet Zlatohlavek. Cromwell stated:

When we got our master's, Roody hadn't started all her neurological research. You see she was an OT then. She had worked in Indianapolis for Winifred Kahmann at Riley's Children [Hospital]. Her housemate, and subsequent chairman of the PT Department at USC, Charlotte Anderson, had also worked for Winnie Kahmann, so that was the source of their clinical skills. Well, she was a marvelous girl.

There are lots of jokes about her. She was a terrible teacher, and that's what most people probably remember, because she had so many ideas, and it came in so many directions that everybody would say, what did Roody teach us today? She taught the stuff to us, but we didn't really know what she was getting at. She never wrote; there was never any writing. She never locked herself down. She didn't have the discipline for that kind of doing, she thought by word of mouth. (Cromwell/Peters oral history, April 28–29, 2003, lines 6,874–6,906; 5,576–5,580; 913–960; 7,479–7,484; 7,544–7,555)

Yerxa reflected:

She was the chairman [USC OT program], in fact she was the one who interviewed me about getting into the program. She was an OT and a

PT. She was very much involved in her own treatment approach, which was using brushing and icing: very physical. So, I'm sure that had an influence on the content of the program. She got so involved in the nervous system, utilizing this external stimulation to produce responses in children that they could produce in a long term way. She was unbelievable; she was absolutely the most unbelievable person because she was a cauldron of energy, a gray-haired whirlwind. (Yerxa/Peters oral history, April 21–22, 2003, lines 513–547; 574–581)

Rood presents an interesting outsider story, an occupational and physical therapist, ostracized by both disciplines. Similar to Ayres, who faced occupational therapy criticism, these women stood their ground and changed occupational therapy's course. Besides their theoretical contributions, their work brought occupational therapy into external debates with other professions. Neuropsychologists, special educators, and physical therapists became aware of emerging occupational therapy theories. Adding this dimension meant occupational therapists broadened their audience beyond physicians.

Mary Reilly

Mary Reilly's theoretical framework, Occupational Behavior, examines how a person's skills, knowledge, and attitudes make functioning possible in life roles (Reilly, 1966). Reilly brought a broader social science perspective to occupational therapy theory, going beyond a pathology mode. Following Rood as a faculty member at USC, Reilly supervised graduate students who are now recognized as contemporary occupational therapy thinkers like Gary Kielhofner and Janice Burke.

Writing perhaps one of the most quoted Eleanor Clarke Slagle lectureships entitled "Occupational therapy can be one of the great ideas of 20th century medicine," in 1961, she asked; "Is occupational therapy a sufficiently vital and unique service for medicine to support and society to reward?" This question reflects occupational therapy's connection to medicine, as an adjunctive support service, rather than a bona fide profession, in the 1960s. Answering her question about occupational therapy's uniqueness, Reilly stated her hypothesis and also her evidence of proof was "that man, through the use of his hands, as they are energized by mind and will, can influence the state of his own health," (Reilly, 1962, p. 2). Fidler identified these words as uplifting for occupational therapy; "I thought that was a beautiful quote," (Fidler/Peters oral history March 6–7, 2003, line 5,167). Bing, while preparing his own Slagle lecture, remembered Reilly's words and stated:

> Once I got over the euphoria of being selected [as a Slagle lecturer], I got busy thinking about a topic. I went back and looked at the previous

lecturers and their topics, and the times in which they delivered them. There was a pattern of sorts. The 'better' ones spoke to an issue of the times; they pushed us at least one step forward. They were believable, in that we expected Betty Yerxa to say pretty much what she said. We expected Willie West to address something current. The one that surprised me most was Mary Reilly. The story is that Willard and Spackman took Mary for a walk around the hotel after she had been selected and before it was announced. They tried to talk her out of it because they felt she was far too controversial. Good old Mary held her ground and delivered probably the most quoted lecture of all.(Bing/Peters oral history, May 3, 2003, lines 1,408–1,416)

Reilly's words "man through the use of his hands..." are familiar to today's occupational therapists and make me wonder why this therapist with inner-circle friendships chose the outsider path, detaching herself from the profession. And what controversy did old guard member Willard fear? Reilly's peer, Wiemer, believes her isolation is more than her wish for retirement, and shared her thoughts stating:

There's a giant hole in our history because she was one of the major factors. She grew a whole generation of practitioners, and without her side of the story it will be unbalanced. I don't know how to deal with it because apparently the Californians themselves can't get access to her. We sorely need it [Reilly's opinion], antagonistic as it may be; we need her concepts of what's going on.

She was incredible. Willie was close; she would vacation with her, and sailed with her, all that kind of thing. She would come to conference, Scottsdale for example, she would come with a stack of books that high. She would sit and read in her room, three books a day, and read book after book after book. She very often would come to conference and never to any meetings. And then she would join various people for lunch or dinner or something, and pick up on what was going on in conference, and made her comments.

Well, there was a time when she was more active, interactive. But in later years, she didn't like all the nonsense of board meetings, all the administrative nonsense. It's a shame Zlatohlavek, her housemate, got sick and died. (Brunyate Wiemer/Peters oral history, March 18–19, 2003, lines 4,990–5,020; 5,044–5,083)

Llorens agreed with Wiemer's concern about losing dissonant scholarly occupational therapy voices and raised questions about Reilly's and other outsider theorists' community acceptance:

Well, I don't know if this has to do with the timing or the abruptness of it, but I think Mary Reilly is a very bright woman. I think she had some brilliant ideas about occupational therapy. And I've been in workshops in which she was participating, when she was still participating. But I believe that she withdrew intellectually from the discourse, if you will. I think the profession loses out when people do that.

I think that's what happened with the Mary Reilly years. I don't think she's ever articulated it the way that I just did. But I think that's why she's been angry for so long, because people don't give credit. They don't give it to anybody. It's not just her or me or Ayres or anybody. When they [AOTA and/or AOTF implied] put together a commission or a committee, like the Philosophical Statement, they don't generally then reference it. (Llorens/ Peters oral history, April 25–26, 2003, lines 5,728–5,743, 6,677–6,694)

Nedra Gillette, Director of Research at AOTF, remembered Reilly fearing misinterpretation. Reilly refused Gillette's formal interview requiring audio-taping for a West-supported foundation project. Gillette stated:

Mary Reilly, we are indebted to her. When I started the oral history interviews a few years ago, since she is such a close friend of Willie's, Willie contacted Mary and said what a nice project this was, and that I was looking forward to interviewing her. So I get out there with my handy little tape recorder to discover that Mary has a grudge against AOTA. Never mind that I'm not representing AOTA, that this was foun-dation project, but she has a grudge against AOTA. (Gillette/Peters inter-view, January 29, 2003, lines 1,959–2,025)

Coming from a blue-collar, Irish–Catholic, Boston family, born in 1916, a girl among brothers, Reilly started at the Boston School. She was not like her classmates Welles and West, who graduated from tony private colleges. In the late 1930s the Boston School of Occupational Therapy had some classes with six students; therefore students knew each other well. Reilly, graduated in 1940, started a lifelong friendship with West and Welles, which is talked about in the following dialogue:

Cromwell: She went to the Boston School when Willie and Carlotta were there; they both had bachelor degrees already, Willie from Holyoke and Carlotta from Scripps. Mary didn't have a bache-lor's yet. She was in the diploma program there.

Welles: She was still a student when I was a student. She had to stay a year longer. When I was in the Boston School, she came back for a third year, and she was around school.

Cromwell: But she was a Boston girl; what's that famous school in Boston? She always was proud that she graduated from, like a church school, but it isn't.[17] She was a good IrishCatholic; they were a good IrishCatholic family. She had lots of broth-ers and they helped in the rug business and lobster business, and things like that. I never heard her speak of her dad. She's older than you are Carlotta, what was she doing beforehand? Mary, she'll be 87 this year and you're only 85.

Welles: I don't know why Mary didn't go to college. Now Willie and the rest of us did. Maybe she couldn't afford it; she was a Catholic. No, but there weren't, I don't know, there weren't...

Cromwell: You're sounding like a Boston elitist or something. (Cromwell/ Welles and Peters oral history, April 28–29, 2003, lines 3,054– 3,060; 5,284–5,354)

An experienced therapist, treating children with cerebral palsy and soldiers with brain injuries early in her career, Reilly continued her education. She was particularly interested in neurology. Earning a Bachelor of Science degree from the University of Southern California in 1951, a Master of Arts degree from San Francisco State College (later University) in 1955, and her Education Doctorate degree (EdD) from the University of California Los Angeles in 1959, Reilly was one of a handful of therapists who received a doctorate in the late 1950s. Bing stated:

I did not know Mary Reilly in those early years. She was a product of the US Army and got her doctorate one year before I did. Then she got interested in play, etc. and eventually took on the graduate program at USC." (Bing/Peters oral history, February 22, 2003, lines 647–650)

Reilly was in with the US Army Medical Department from 1941 to 1955. During the war years, Reilly worked in the Service Command Surgeon's Office, Fourth Service Command, in Atlanta, Georgia from 1944 to 1946. Supervising occupational therapy services at 20 military hospitals, she received the Meritorious Civilian Service Award. This military history influenced future career experiences, like funding her own graduate education, and facilitating master's research work for numerous military occupational therapists at USC.

Reilly continued USC's OT think-tank tradition, working closely with Rood's succeeding chair, Harriet Zlatohlavek. Forming a life-long professional and private partnership, Reilly and Zlatohlavek were housemates. Reilly officially retired in 1977 from USC as a Professor Emeritus. Zlatohlavek, or Miss Harriet as students called her, and Reilly kept USC's occupational therapy department afloat in the 1960s and 1970s with grant and research funding. Federal level funding came from the Maternal and Child Health Service in the Department of Health, Education and Welfare (HEW) where colleague and close friend Willie West held the position of occupational therapy consultant. Reilly (1974) acknowledged this connection in the preface to her book, *Play As Exploratory Learning*, thanking West for financial support and for encouraging her in the completion of the text. Cromwell remembered the 1970s at USC and stated:

Tough years that Harriet maneuvered through. We survived on MCH grants because Willie was very good to us. They had been friends for eons, Mary and Willie. They were all BSOTs. But they did army together, and see Mary was army too. Mary and Willie were the assistants to Winifred Kahmann, who ran the army occupational therapy service. (Cromwell/Peters oral history, April 28–29, 2003, lines 7,682–7,695)

Cromwell continued to talk about the time that she held the position of USC OT chair following Zlatohlavek and said:

Well, I was there as kind of the undergirding to help it work because Mary was obviously the think machine in what we did with the students. Helping us get kids with the behaviors (referring to Reilly's Occupational Behavior frame of reference) and understanding that what they needed was not just learning how to weave and how they do woodwork, and how to measure range of motion and so on. Cromwell/Peters oral history, April 28–29, 2003, lines 7,402–7,411)

Similarly, Yerxa remembered taking over the USC OT curriculum and discovering Reilly's departmental papers. She stated:

See when I went to SC in '76 she [Reilly] had left in '75. I inherited a lot of stuff she had worked on. That's really when I began to respect what she had done, because she didn't write that much. But when I saw the master's theses that had come out under her direction, and when I saw how they had structured the curriculum, I thought, wow this is powerful stuff here.

They did use activity analysis, but it was from a very broad perspective, which involved the developmental level of the individual. It involved psychological factors and cultural factors. All of the things that I was talking about with an integral science, now that I think about it. Yes they did activity analysis, but it was more like what the potential effects of this activity might have on the various components of the human being, not just a cause/effect relationship.

I don't know if you've ever read *Play as Exploratory Learning*,[18] which to me is the heart of everything. I used to use that in graduate seminar; it was so rich, but extremely difficult because she does not spell things out. You have to know a lot, you have to read a lot to know some of the things she's saying. But the book is interesting, because the whole book is about pathology, not about intervention, it's about play and the human spirit, and how significant it is about what we become. And then she had all of her graduate students do the pathology part. The application; that was the applied [science]. And the same with Ayres in Sensory Integration, so I think that's quite fascinating. (Yerxa/Peters oral history, April 21–22, 2003, lines 3,829–3,850, 4,327–4,351)

Llorens also spoke about that time and said:

Mary Reilly, Mary Reilly's work, see Mary didn't publish, she pontificated.[19] And the people who were closest to her heard the things that she had to say, and her students heard what she had to say. The Occupational Behavior [frame of reference] was what she was talking about, and I think most of the publications were by other people later on. But it wasn't being published, so it wasn't out there. I wasn't a part of that inner circle [referring to USC], so I didn't know what they were doing. In some ways it validated what we were thinking [referring to Llorens' theoretical work and research in child and adolescent mental health], if there were some parallels. And there were some parallels. (Llorens/ Peters oral history, April 25–26, 2003, lines 2,428–2,471)

Mary Reilly, a thinker and avid reader, gathered her theoretical work from broad sources beyond the hard sciences, including philosophy, sociology, anthropology, psychology, and other social sciences. It also came from her psychiatric clinical work starting in the 1940s. Fidler spiritedly remembered first meeting Reilly and their intellectual sparring and stated:

All along, all along we argued and argued. When she was in Boston, I was there at some kind of meeting and met her for the first time. Immediately we were engaged in an argument and that continued. Then she was in the Army, and I was in the Army, and then we also argued. I used to accuse her of ambiguities; she said one thing and did another. She'd chide me with my concern about the symbolic meaning of activities.

She'd say 'That's nothing, that's nothing;'' she didn't think the unconscious existed. Right, she had trouble, she didn't like the unconscious at all, and I was very much focused on the unconscious. I was in analysis and all of that. So we were coming from very different perspectives. I used to say, 'I acknowledge that, but we have to look at the dimensions of meaning, there are symbolic messages as well'. 'Well, that's not my cup of tea,' she'd say. So that was an argument that went on and on, time and time again. (Fidler/Peters oral history, March 6–7, 2003, lines 5,102–5,156)

The community of therapists knew about Reilly and Fidler's oil and water mix. Nedra Gillette, a University of Illinois occupational therapy graduate, talked about how community insider and Program Director Wade instructed her to make plans for a Reilly and Fidler encounter at a 1960s American Medical Association (AMA) meeting. She stated:

When I was still teaching in Illinois in the mid '60s, there was an AMA conference in Chicago. Bea Wade worked with AOTA to make sure they had a representative at AMA. The AOTA sent Gail Fidler and Mary Reilly to this conference. Bea called me into her office and said 'You're going to be on duty this week along with me. It's our job to keep these two women apart so that the AMA has the benefit of what they both have to offer, but that they don't get into some great big horrendous fight.' I said, 'That's quite an assignment.' She said 'Never mind, that's what we're going to do.' So Bea and I spent the weekend with Mary and Gail, and there was no fighting. There were some humorous remarks. They both represented the profession magnificently in what they had to say about what occupational therapy could offer to the field of mental health. (Gillette/Peters interview, Jan 29, 2003, lines 2,031–2,060)

Reilly, opinionated at times, didn't hesitate to express her thoughts using clear and colorful language. When AOTA leader, Fidler, campaigned for a politically difficult undertaking to include the creative arts therapies (art, music, and dance) under a potential occupational therapy umbrella in the 1960s, Reilly vehemently opposed the proposition. Fidler remembered Reilly's comments and said: "You know she made me furious when she said, 'You lie down with dogs, you come up with fleas.' I said I thought that was a pompous, arrogant statement, unworthy of herself or anyone else. Oh, I was furious." (Fidler/Peters oral history March 6–7, 2003, lines 5,156–5,161) If successful, this professional amalgamation would have broadened occupational therapy's jurisdiction and powerbase (Abbott, 1988). Fidler remembered Reilly standing her ground, wanting an unadulterated occupational therapy, or one without other disciplines. Taking this a step further, Reilly viewed occupational therapy as superior to other therapies, rather than lesser. Fidler also believed in occupational therapy's worth but strategized differently from Reilly.

The community understood and accepted Reilly's theoretical contributions and ability to think. They also understood her exclusiveness and peppery opinions. The next scholar, Anne Mosey, who was younger than Ayres, Rood, and Reilly, also held an outsider community position in occupational therapy's history.

Anne C. Mosey

Mosey, contributing to occupational therapy theoretical knowledge in the 1970s, conceptualized three frames of references: analytical, acquisitional, and developmental (Mosey, 1981, 1986; Hopkins, 1978). These frames of reference provided a guideline for occupational therapy psychiatric practice that differed from other theories. Her 1960s group process analysis work came from her own experiences as a clinician and her interest in sociology and psychology (Mosey, 1973).

Mosey conceptualized a taxonomy or configuration for occupational therapy knowledge. Her career-long study of occupational therapy knowledge culminated in her 1990 work, *Epistemological Orientations of Practice*, described in Section I. Like the ideas of her peers, Mosey's work provided a theoretical rationale for occupational therapy intervention, thus broadening and bringing new scholarship to the profession and ultimately to patients.

Her analytic framework addressed peoples' need for fulfillment. The acquisitional framework addressed a person's environmental interactions based upon skills and abilities. Finally, linked to the acquisitional, the developmental framework discussed the maturational stages required for people to interact in their larger community. Llorens, an occupational therapy developmental theorist, talked about studying occupational therapy literature when she was preparing her own Slagle lecture in the following quotation. As Llorens stated, she remembered Mosey's theoretical work in the late 1960s, and put occupational therapy's theory development into the context of the times. She said:

> Oh, Mosey. At that time I think she was the only one talking about adaptation in the way we [the interdisciplinary team at the Lafayette Clinic in Michigan] were talking about mastery and that sort of thing. That would probably have been why I have selected her [theoretical work]. She's gone off on some other directions, but this was '69.
>
> Gail Fidler influenced the work that was more related to projective techniques, and that sort of thing. But in terms of theory at that time . . . I I don't think so in terms of occupational therapy. We didn't have occupational therapists who were pure scientists in relationship to behavior. The occupational therapists, as I recall, were more focused on techniques, and to some extent outcomes. Well, it wasn't outcome in the way that it is today. I mean results, results of therapy. But it wasn't theoretically grounded. And I do think that since you've asked me the question, and I'm thinking about it that Anne Mosey was one of the first people who had written some things on theory. I'm trying to think, I was not aware of theoretical things coming out of Southern California other than Jean Ayres. (Llorens/Peters oral history, April 25–26, lines 2,352–2,423)

Gail Fidler, early career mentor to Mosey, an isolated scholar, introduced her to the community of therapists. From 1961 until 1966 Mosey worked at the New York State Psychiatric Institute in New York City under Fidler's supervision. Fidler talked about Mosey and her place as an occupational therapy scholar. She stated:

> I would say that Anne Mosey is a scholar. You may not like her style, but she's a scholar. Anne Mosey, she was a recalcitrant. She has always been very generous about me, and acknowledged me as a mentor. She'll say that, but there are logic tight compartments in her head. She's very bright. I think of the special relationship I had with Anne Mosey, the difficulties, the problems, and also her smarts and her capabilities. And working through [them] in order to . . . and that's another part of my philosophy that really is the basis of my lifestyle performance model, to use her strengths rather than focus on her weaknesses. To use her strengths, I see it in that way, she's using her strengths. She's the one who's doing that, not me. (Fidler/Peters oral history, March 6–7, 2003, lines 4,066–4,079; 2,763–2,809)

Gilfoyle, talking about occupational therapy's inner circle, spoke about Mosey's independence and said:

> Anne didn't want to do that [be part of the inner circle]. She was more a rebel; she was her own person. She believed what she believed and she was doing her own thing. I think that's why I always admired her.
>
> I think back, and it seems to me she may have called me on the phone to talk to me about working with Slack [publishing house] and the contract [publication process]. I think it was on the phone and not at a conference. Questions about what do I do about royalties, and how did you find them about marketing your book. It was nice; she would reach out to people. I can't remember if our books came out at the same time. I remember being very impressed by her book and using it. (Gilfoyle/Peters oral history, February 10–11, 2003, lines 3,069–3,092)

Following her initial career working in psychiatry, Mosey briefly taught at Columbia University and later New York University where she developed occupational therapy's first Doctor of Philosophy degree in the 1970s. Similar to Reilly, Mosey taught today's occupational therapy scholars and leaders like Clark and Hinojosa. Mosey continued fitting the community outsider profile as noted by one author, Menks Ledwig, who said, "no one seemed to understand what she was talking about, thus experiencing subsequent lack of support" (1988, p. 44). Community member Marion Crampton remembered Mosey teaching theory to occupational therapy assistants. Mosey provided consultation services from 1966 to1969 for the Vocational Rehabilitation Act–Occupational Therapy Assistant (VRA–OTA) Project for the Massachusetts Department of Mental Health. Crampton stated "Somehow I got a grant to write something that was suitable for OT assistants for teaching. Anne Mosey did it. She did the writing of the book. Of course it was way over everybody's heads" (Crampton/Peters oral history, March 1, 2003, lines 1,128–1,135).

It is not clear whether Mosey chose her outsider status or whether a core group of insiders excluded her based on her thoughts and behaviors. There are questions about occupational therapy sisterhood and what it is based on. These questions go beyond how therapists functioned among themselves. The larger question is this: What organizational purpose did this dissonant group of theorists serve in developing this profession? Outsider theorists challenged a well-ingrained status quo and broke new ground. Insiders, old-guard sustainers in particular, supported a compliant tradition, historically working closely with physicians. Recalcitrant community outsiders asked the hard questions and harshly criticized occupational therapy's validity. In so doing, these therapists made scholarly strides and changed occupational therapy.

Insider Theorists

Gail Fidler and Elizabeth Yerxa were futurists, representing different generations. Fidler's career spanned more than 65 years, and Yerxa's 50 years. Both
women were grounded in thoughts about occupational therapy's potential,
but had differing perspectives. Yerxa used words like "audacious," "seductive,"
and "provocative" in describing occupational therapy. Fidler ardently challenged occupational therapy to the membership and to the profession, and
saw her years spent in promoting the profession as exhausting. She said
"I think, finally after all these years, I'm getting burned out. I'm tired of saying
'god damn.' I think our sense of inadequacy really precludes exploration,
because not knowing, we see that as a negative" (Fidler/Peters oral history,
March 6–7, 2003, lines 789–815). Although each holds different views and
comes from opposite sides of the country, Fidler's and Yerxa's common
denominator is the determination which catapulted occupational therapy forward. For example, Fidler's 1965 Slagle lecture presented the argument that
occupational therapy has the responsibility to develop a framework and body
of knowledge for professional education. Yerxa's 1966 Slagle lecture talked
about "authentic" occupational therapy, challenging therapists to own and
revere the profession's uniqueness and expanding body of knowledge. Both
addresses provided a framework for professionalization.

Gail S. Fidler

Joining Gail Fidler (1916–2005) in her Florida sunroom, the first thing I saw
next to her favorite chair was a low bookcase filled with the 13 occupational
therapy books she had authored. There were no occupational therapy
awards displayed, although she had received the respected Eleanor Clarke
Slagle Lectureship in 1965, the Award of Merit in 1980, and in 2002 was
the 8th recipient of AOTA and AOTF's The President's Commendation in
honor of Wilma L. West. (AOTF Connection, Summer 2002c, p. 4) Rather,
her books silently displayed her career legacy. She identified her first book
fondly, *Introduction to Psychiatric Occupational Therapy*, co-authored with
her psychiatrist husband, Jay W. Fidler, in 1954. The cornerstone book in
psychiatric occupational therapy for its time, the Fidler's broke new conceptual ground. Well accepted by community insiders, Fidler, remembering, said
"The only accolades I ever received were when I published my first book. I
had a large stack of letters and notes saying this is wonderful" (Fidler/Peters
oral history, March 6–7, 2003, lines 5,895–5,898). Her professional partnership with Jay Fidler and former supervisor, Arthur P. Noyes, MD, Superin-
tendent of the Norristown State Hospital and American Psychiatric
Association President in 1955, provided intellectual sparing. It also gave
Fidler the opportunity to explain occupational therapy's worth to other

professionals, leading to her writing about the multidisciplinary team (Fidler 1957, 1981, 1983).

Throughout her career, Fidler explored symbolic meaning, designing activity laboratories, including projective tasks such as clay and finger paints, or physical activities that assessed and engaged psychiatric patients. Known for *Doing and becoming*, the Fidlers (1978) discussed self-actualization through purposeful activities. Continually searching for rationales, she analyzed the meaning of activity, developing her Lifestyle Performance Profile in the 1980s. The lifestyle performance profile (Fidler, 1982) is an acquisitional frame of reference describing how sustaining health depends upon achieving critical skill clusters, including self-care, meeting self-needs, intrinsic gratification, and service to others. Doing or engaging in purposeful activity is seen as the essence of learning and adaptation. Fidler identified this frame of reference as a "product of pragmatism in contrast to theoretical research," (Fidler, 1988, p. 39). This statement illustrates her thoughts about her "hands on" approach to occupational therapy intervention.

Fidler, a strong individualist, entered her career and marriage equal to her husband. Together they formed one of the strongest unions promoting occupational therapy's merits, particularly in psychiatry. A community insider finding few peers other than Elizabeth (Betty) Ridgway, Marion Crampton in her early psychiatric career, and a long friendship with insider Wilma West, Fidler spoke about her being ahead of her time and stated:

> I promoted occupational therapy in the context and meaning that nobody else understood. That was a very lonely place to be; I could find no companions. I need the stimulation of other people thinking and I want people to argue with me. Sometimes it was very scary . . . is this the right limb that I am sitting on or not? Of course, that's what risk is all about, and with no risk, there is no growth. (Fidler/Peters oral history, March 6–7, 2003, lines 7,557–7,577; 4,339–4,351).

Fidler entered the community after being graduated from the Philadelphia School under old-guard insider Helen Willard. Fidler, a non-conformist, remembered Willard at the Philadelphia School and said:

> If I had a mentor, it was Helen Willard, which is surprising because I argued with her every day of my life. I made her life miserable most of the time. I couldn't fit the protocol. I'm sure I drove her up the wall and back down. We wore these horrible green uniforms with white collars and starched cuffs. I would take the cuffs off, roll up my sleeves and be chastised for being out of uniform. Or, I would forget my cuffs and then there would be a call from Helen Willard's office. She would say 'Now Miss Spangle, you left your white cuffs,' and she would shake

her finger at me. I would tell her that her white cuffs were nonsense. She'd say 'You have to accept some rules and regulations,' I'd say, 'Well not white cuffs.' We'd argue about those damn things forever. (Fidler/Peters oral history, March 6–7, 2003, lines 436–480)

Fidler openly and honestly questioned her career choice. Prior to entering occupational therapy, Fidler decided against an elementary school teaching career. After finishing her occupational therapy certificate at the Philadelphia School, she said:

I remember when I left school and entered practice, I was shocked! I said, 'My God, have I chosen the wrong career? This is not what I expected, if this is the way it is.' I did my typical problem solving process. I said 'If this is the way it is, I'm going to try to change it; I'll give myself one year. I'll keep notes and if it's not better, I'll quit and go someplace else. I'll leave OT.' (Fidler/Peters oral history, March 6–7, 2003, lines 696–705)

When questioned about what brought her to occupational therapy, Fidler described various motivators. Two things stand out in her answers. First, that she didn't enter occupational therapy to help people like her peers Crampton, Gilfoyle, Llorens, Stattel, Wiemer, and Yerxa did. Second, that she entered at a time when women had limited professional options. About this, she said:

Well, I think that my reason for entering OT is different from, in all probability, anybody else's. I think that accounts for some of the diversity of my interests. I was interested and curious about activities and what they meant. That's what I cared about; I didn't enter to help people, to be useful or anything else. I was curious about how activities relate to human behavior. (Fidler/Peters oral history, March 6–7, 2003, lines 5–26)

Having limited financial resources, Fidler said she was not able to pursue medicine, a difficult path for women in the early 1940s. She explained that occupational therapy was her road to psychiatry and said:

It was the constraints of society; medicine wasn't open to women. I wasn't prepared; I didn't have the money to fight it. That was another reason for going into OT, to get enough experience and credentials to move into medicine. OT was a jumping point, and it would give me information about the questions I asked. I was interested in psychiatry because I felt that would give me better leverage, finding out what I wanted as a physician in psychiatry rather than as an OT. (Fidler/Peters oral history, March 6–7, 2003, lines 1,531–1,550)

Fidler balked at gender boundaries, financial challenges, and societal constraints. These feelings were related to her upbringing. Some of her views came from her progressive father, a high school physical education teacher. Similar to other community members, Fidler's father challenged her thinking. About this she said:

> We were very poor. My father was a high school teacher. He would have dug ditches in order to enable us to go to college. I was my father's son. He was the most important person in my learning and growing up. He taught me that argument was one of the best ways of learning. He was a taskmaster, and a difficult man in many ways. 'Don't be a pussyfoot,' or, 'What are you, a little mouse? Stand up and say what it is you think.' He would bring to the dinner table a provocative statement, and I would rise to the bait. I was fortunate that my father molded me into a different kettle of fish. I was always free to make up my own mind. I don't think I ever set out to be different, it just was. I relied on my thinking. I was always curious; I always wanted to know why. (Fidler/Peters oral history, March 6–7, 2003, lines 2,964–2,965; 2,995–2,996; 2,827–2,865; 3,722; 4,761–4,777; 4,950–4,955; 6,962–6,975; 7,161–7,163; 2,950–2,952)

Learning that she could use her thinking abilities to break gender and career barriers, Fidler, a wife for more than 50 years, and the mother of two children, questioned traditional roles. Resistant to her mother's modeling, she made her career a priority; spending months commuting to various positions, and returning home weekends. Having a career starting in the early 1940s, she went down her own path. She stated:

> I was not a typical woman in the 50 s. I was not a typical woman in the 30 s. The influence that my mother had on me was for me to demonstrate I was not going to end up being like my mother who was bright and capable, but did very little, if anything, about it. I was not going to be a laid-back compliant woman, giving her all for her husband and her children. That was my mother's role, to take care of my father, and take care of her children. My brother was retarded; he had brain damage when he was about 7, so her whole life was around him. (Fidler/Peters oral history, March 6–7, 2003, lines 187–192, 3,008–3,020)

Fidler spoke about how balancing career and family was not easy, particularly when she accepted employment away from the family. She said:

> It was never easy. I struggled all the time with a sense of guilt; you know you just do. The contract I had with myself was that I had to earn enough money to pay a full-time nanny and housekeeper so that I always had someone living in I could trust and value. When I went to AOTA he [her husband, Jay Fidler] was home in New Jersey and I went to

Washington. I came home on the weekends if I wasn't on the West Coast. I would drive 400 miles one way. He did his thing and I did my thing, and that's the way we operated all along. (Fidler/Peters, oral history, March 6–7, 2003, lines 3,106–3,125; 3,650–3,660)

Fidler, a community insider, saw herself as different and not well-understood. This self-perception also belies the notion of a well-integrated occupational therapy sisterhood. Did other community insiders feel isolated and different? This question presents an interesting paradox, considering that these people were progressive leaders and individualistic thinkers. Fidler identified herself as different or ahead of her time. She talked about isolation and career struggles. An accomplished administrator working in the New Jersey mental health system, her AOTA career did not go the way she wanted it to. Fidler held the title of both interim and associate executive director of AOTA in the early 1970s during Cromwell's presidency. Following the difficulty finding a replacement for Tiebel, Leo Fanning, a non-occupational therapist, accepted the post in 1972. Fidler, holding an AOTA administrative position, clashed with Fanning. After his exit, Fidler was the interim executive director. This position later became associate executive director under James Garibaldi, a non-therapist retired Navy officer, who was originally brought on to monitor budgetary issues. Fidler wanted the executive director position that eventually fell to Garibaldi and spoke about her career upset and community betrayal. About this she said:

I wanted to retain that position very badly [interim executive director], because I felt like I could do a lot to shape up AOTA and the profession. I was obviously too strong. I believe the central office should be a leader in the development of a profession. The board and AOTA membership seemingly believed that it should be the president, which is ridiculous, because every three years you change direction to fit the new president. Nobody ever agreed with me on that. I was angry and frustrated, and I had devoted too much time and energy to develop the damn thing! (Fidler/Peters oral history, March 6–7, 2003, lines 2,393–2,445)

Gillette, then AOTA Secretary, remembered the executive director search and said:

We had a search committee, which as secretary I was asked to chair. I knew nothing about this; I had never played big-league ball. Gail Fidler, Lyla Spelbring, and I met and talked about what we wanted in the way of an executive director. We looked at all the recommendations that were flowing into us from around the country. Gail was very interested, but I think the board was not ready for her maverick type of leadership at the time. What the three of us concluded and presented to the board was to open the search to outsiders who had experience in health care administration. We would make Gail the associate executive director for practice, education and research. Then we would have an associate executive director for business and finance. (Gillette/Peters oral history, January 29, 2003, lines 788–818)

Gillette's remembrances illustrate how Fidler was a community insider, participating in AOTA decision-making alongside established insider, Spelbring, yet not fully supported.

Fidler, acknowledging her controversial style, considered her insider and outsider status dichotomy, seeing herself as too progressive for more conservative community leaders. About this she stated:

> I think that I'm about 10 years ahead, because what I said 12 years ago is now beginning to be looked at. It's over their heads. I am always out there at the end of the pole by myself. When I received that award recently from the Foundation and AOTA, the President's Award, I said that one of the things that had been said about me was that I was 10 years ahead of the game. That could be and was a very lonely position. You're out there, and you don't find anybody who agrees with you. (Fidler/Peters oral history, March 6–7, 2003, lines 5,914–5,918; 1,414–1,426)

Fidler is not the only community member who identified herself as ahead of her time. In many ways arguments can be made for all the community members that I studied as being progressive in their own way. Fidler is unique in bridging the gap between old-guard and newer community members, mentoring other Slagle recipients like Anne C. Mosey and Susan B. Fine,[20] three who received their lectureship awards in the mid-1980s and early 1990s, respectively, while remaining outspoken.

Elizabeth J. Yerxa

Elizabeth Yerxa, known as Betty to her peers, is one of occupational therapy's most comprehensive thinkers and promoters of research (AOTF, 1983). She is also a community of therapist insiders, theorist, and futurist. Remaining an active scholar, teaching, and consulting abroad and in this country, she characterizes herself as an isolated thinker. When I questioned her about her thinking style, Yerxa responded:

> I would say I'm an independent thinker, very much so. Not to say that I haven't been influenced by others, but I think that most of the real hard thinking that I've done has been independent. I like nothing better than to sit and try to synthesize the reading I've been doing and apply it to the field. I do that all the time. I think, how does this apply to occupational therapy or occupational therapy science?[21] (Yerxa/Peters oral history, April 21–22, 2003, lines 3,142–3,156; 360–367)

Yerxa characterized herself as a voracious reader drawn to philosophy. By combining these interests, she has written about an occupational therapy philosophical base. (Yerxa, 1979; 1983; 1992)

> I read constantly. I'm drawn to philosophy, so I'm more likely to read in that area. I've always loved to write; it probably goes back to junior high school. I found it quite easy to write, if it was the right time and subject. (Yerxa/Peters oral history, April 21–22, 2003, lines 360–367; 3,029–3,032)

Understandably, she appeared at home in her bookcase-lined living room in her mountaintop house with its panoramic view of California's pristine high desert country. Her scholarly and leadership contributions span her 50-year career. A continuing theme of her career, stated in Yerxa's Slagle lecture and throughout her writings, was strong encouragement of therapists to own and act upon occupational therapy's authenticity as a true profession. Other community members like West, Wiemer, Fidler, Gilfoyle, and Cromwell shared this concern, putting professionalism on occupational therapy's radar screen. Gilfoyle shared her thoughts about Yerxa's role in promoting occupational therapy and stated:

> I think she [Yerxa] was quite instrumental in the profession. She is a little older than I, but she was so involved. There was a real movement with people like Mary Reilly, Jean Ayres, and even Ann [Grady] and I, to grab hold of what occupational therapy was about. Betty Yerxa was the real key. (Gilfoyle/Peters oral history, February 10–11, 2003, lines 1,198–1,208)

Similarly, when Yerxa received her University of Southern California Distinguished Professor Emeritus honor, West (1991) described Yerxa's contributions and stated, "Scholar, theorist, philosopher, educator, researcher, mentor, teacher—all these terms and more are appropriate characterizations of the many roles Betty Yerxa has played during her distinguished career as an OT. One wishes she could be cloned again and again (Tapper, 1991, OT Week, April 4, p. 2)." Yerxa identified her commitment to occupational therapy as a drive and even as an awakening when she first discovered occupational therapy as a high school student. About this she stated:

> What I knew about OT, that was it, that "Aha!" experience. I was motivated by humanistic values. I wanted to really help people. I think I felt frustrated by being put in a small box, about what OT is and what OT could be. I always felt so committed to the profession that I felt strongly about issues. I think that was the motivation to write instead of just letting it be a turmoil inside of me. A lot of the writing that I had done, particularly editorials, have been out of a real sense of feeling for the profession. (Yerxa/Peters oral history, April 21–22, 2003, lines 4,676–4,677; 1,062–1,066; 3,035–3,043)

Yerxa continues to contribute to the occupational therapy's scientific and philosophical knowledge base, as part of her career-long belief that occupational therapy is a bona fide profession. This is illustrated in her 1966 Slagle lecture in which she stated:

> Perhaps most significant for the future development of our body of knowledge is the increased awareness that the scientific attitude is not incompatible with concern for the client as a human being, but may be one of the best foundations for acting upon that concern. (Yerxa, 1967a, p. 1)

Breaking tradition, Yerxa was a very young Slagle recipient in 1966, with only 14 years of experience as an occupational therapist. For example, she presented her lecture after more professionally senior community members such as Stattel, Wiemer, Reilly, Ayres, and Fidler, and just before West. She reflected on her career contributions when asked, seeing herself as a scholar and leader. She stated:

> I think today, April 22, 2003, I see myself as a scholar. That is related to the content of what I'm doing, which is reading, writing, thinking, and presenting from time to time. In the past, I probably would have characterized myself as a professional leader. I don't think that I've ever forgotten my roots in practice. My work at AOTA and AOTF—it was more leadership in terms of the direction of the profession. I've had my foot in various camps. (Yerxa/Peters oral history, April 21–22, 2003, lines 4,083–4,094; 4,105–4,112)

Her community entrance came through her contributions and academic pedigree. A University of California graduate in 1952, she met community members Rood, when Yerxa was still a young practitioner, Cromwell and Welles while she was on internship at Los Angeles County Hospital, and West while West was on campus pursuing her advanced master's degree. Talking about discovering occupational therapy at the University of Southern California, Yerxa remembered:

> When I was in high school I could not decide on a career objective because my interests were so broad. I wanted to find something that encompassed everything, but it also had to have some science. I was interested in science, in the arts, in psychology and human factors. I read this article in Seventeen Magazine, and it described this profession called occupational therapy. It had pictures of OTs working with patients. I had gone through, as you did in those days, counseling in high school about professions. They'd say social work or film directing, but no one ever mentioned occupational therapy. I don't think they knew enough about it then; it was back in the 40s. I got a scholarship because I was an academic

overachiever. I started at SC the fall of 1948 and finished in 1952.(Yerxa/
Peters oral history, April 21–22, 2003, lines 4–40; 4,580–4,581; 4,604–4,608)

Drawn to a different learning environment on the East Coast, Yerxa left
California and earned her Master of Education degree in Educational
Psychology in 1968, and shortly afterward earned her Doctor of Education
in Educational Psychology in 1971 at Boston University. There she met community member and controversial outsider Jerry Johnson.[22] Speaking about
those who influenced her thinking, and about earning her doctoral degree
at a time when few did, Yerxa stated:

> I think I was accepted. I may be naïve to say this, and some people prob-
> ably perceived me as a threat. But mainly I felt accepted and felt like
> people thought we're moving in this direction now, having doctoral level
> education. I never thought of leaving the field or doing anything else
> with my doctoral studies. It was moving ahead. I felt I gained a voice
> among other professions as a result of this educational choice.
>   I remember Wilma West's, Mary Reilly's, and Jerry Johnson's
> influence on me. I was never her [Reilly's] student. It was through the
> work she had done at [U]SC which I inherited when I went there as the
> chairman. I knew Jerry when she was the chairman at Boston University
> in the OT program. I had a part-time position teaching there until I
> became a TA in my own doctoral work. (Yerxa/Peters oral history, April
> 21–22, 2003, lines 2,409–2,427; 1,944–1,953; 2,145–2,150)

Yerxa's community entrance and profile as an educated woman earning
degrees from fine private universities gave her opportunities not available to
her parents, who struggled during the 1930s depression like many other
Americans. She learned the value of education at a young age, and both
her parents groomed her and her sister for a university education. She
explained, "Both of my parents, from the time I was this high made it very
clear that I was going to college, there was no way around it. I'm very grate-
ful for that" (Yerxa/Peters oral history, April 21–22, 2003, lines 76–81).
    Always knowing she was university bound, Yerxa discussed her practical
goal of getting a job, a common goal of middle-class, first-generation, college-
educated people. Her goals and values thus differed from the values of some
of her more privileged upper- and middle-class classmates at the University of
Southern California. They and some more affluent community members had
the luxury to study for education's sake. Yerxa reflected:

> I would say I'm from the middle class or even lower-middle class during
> the time we were struggling during the depression. When I think about it,
> I'm lucky I went to SC because my intention in going to school was to pre-
> pare myself for a job. It was very practical, and that's pretty much the way
> we thought about it. I wasn't thinking of it as education with a capitol E, or

[the] preparation for life, or citizenship. When I look back, I envy people who looked at their education in a broader sense, not for job preparation, but for the exploration of ideas. I never felt I had that luxury, versus people like Wilma West and Carlotta Welles, who went to the university to become educated; it was a completely different objective. They were educated for life, not for a job, so I was completely lucky. (Yerxa/Peters oral history, April 21–22, 2003, lines 1,913–1,934; 4,611–4,640)

Yerxa's more practical nature may be rooted in her childhood memories of the depression and her brother's death in World War II. She shared how these more global events shaped her beliefs and stated:

I grew up in LA [Los Angeles], a several-generation Californian. I think my formative experience in my young life was the depression. I was about eight. We had a terrible time; we had no electricity in our house. My parents made it a game, cooking on our fireplace. We couldn't pay the gas bill for our stove. My father came to California to work in the oil fields. He was never able to go to college, even though he was a very bright person. Mother was a very bright person who went to the university one semester but had to quit because of economic reasons. She had been a homemaker, but later worked at Lockheed Aircraft because women were needed as part of the labor force during World War II. I had a brother, the oldest in our family, who was killed in World War II when I was twelve. His death was a shadow over our lives. The depression and the war were very significant in my life. (Yerxa/Peters oral history, April 21–22, 2003, lines 48–95; 116–150)

Similarly to Fidler, Yerxa spoke about dinner table arguments and conversations that stimulated her critical reasoning skills and ability to think. Unlike Fidler's father's thought-provoking questions, Yerxa's parents motivated her and her sister to engage in the discussions. She stated:

We had a very stimulating home environment where we would talk about ideas. We would not only talk, we would argue. We always had to have the facts, and the evidence. We had to be able to defend our position. Both of my parents contributed to that. (Yerxa/Peters oral history, April 21–22, 2003, lines 598–617)

Yerxa further discussed her mother's influence and said:

My mother was very important; I consider her my cheerleader. She always believed in me, and also felt that I could do anything. I think growing up I felt like that; anything I set my mind to, I could do, and that probably was due to my mother. But it wasn't all positive because my mother was very perfectionistic, and I've had problems with that. I feel like I can do anything but I'm very self-critical at the same time. (Yerxa/Peters oral history, April 21–22, 2003, lines 4,367–4,376)

Yerxa generalized the belief that women could do anything they set their minds to, bringing a sense of activism and feminism to occupational therapy. Socially aware, experiencing first-hand activism at Boston University when she was a doctoral student teaching assistant in the late 1960s, Yerxa and close colleague, Johnson, believed in a more progressive occupational therapy. Yerxa, influenced by the 1960s and 1970s human rights and disabilities awareness movements, promoted a socially sensitive and involved occupational therapy. Yerxa's work promoting occupational therapy research and scientific contributions is discussed in Section VI.

This section discussed community groupings including theorists, political movers, and sustainers. These groupings remain fluid because some therapists fall into multiple categories. For example, Fidler can be identified both as a theorist and a political mover. Llorens, characterized as a sustainer in the next section can also be identified as a theorist, as was political mover Gilfoyle. Each grouping served a separate function to occupational therapy's evolution. Most notable was the division between theorists on one side, and political movers and sustainers on the other. They viewed occupational therapy differently, theorists supporting a masculinized science base, and political movers and sustainers supporting a philosophically based occupational therapy. More significant was the covert division that rose from these different vantage points, and how dissonance influenced change. Overt disagreement, not part of occupational therapy culture, was suppressed in the community. Political movers, holding internal control, understood theorists contributions, and rather than splitting occupational therapy, leaders knew that outsiders made contributions that could not be ignored. Therefore, Section V illuminates how the political movers and sustainers functioned, and their beliefs.

SECTION V: POLITICAL MOVERS AND SUSTAINERS

The political movers Ruth Brunyate Wiemer, Florence Cromwell, and Elnora Gilfoyle served as AOTA presidents in the 1960s, 1970s, and the 1980s. Prior to their presidencies, each therapist exemplified leadership, professional commitment, and caring. Seeking the best for occupational therapy, these women with varying personalities responded to the larger membership's needs. Experiencing similar outcomes but different methods, political movers made occupational therapy known to a larger audience.

Good at people connections, political movers were community insiders who worked well with Wilma West. Were these the women who determined occupational therapy's professional direction over all other community factions? How did the political movers change occupational therapy to a science-based profession? Did they prioritize knowledge development, like theorists, or did they consider other matters more pressing, like forming alliances with legislators, or gaining professional autonomy, particularly from medicine?

Ruth Brunyate Wiemer

Ruth Brunyate Wiemer is an energetic, thoughtful woman with a razor-sharp wit who lives on the tranquil banks of the Chester River in Maryland. Wiemer, a community of therapists' insider, characterized herself as shy. A surprising disclosure, considering that she approached government officials in the hallways of the United States Senate and House of Representatives, lobbying for occupational therapy causes in the 1960s and 1970 s. In light of her reserve, she explained how she was able to became one of the profession's strongest spokespersons on Capitol Hill and said, "Basically at heart I'm a rather shy and quiet person. My friends don't believe it but it's true. You see, I had all my peers supporting me, it never was a problem" (Wiemer/Peters oral history, March 18–19, 2003, lines 639–641; 660–661).

Understated and humble about her accomplishments, she talked about her career while sitting in her comfortable Eastern Shore Maryland living room. Receiving occupational therapy's highest honors, her awards included the Eleanor Clarke Slagle lecture in 1957 and the Award of Merit (AOTA, 1969) in 1968 and the Wilma L. West AOTA-AOTF President's Commendation in 1998 (AOTA 1998a). She was the first recipient of the Lindy Boggs award, named after the United States Senator from Louisiana who supported occupational therapy. Wiemer remembered the meaning of the Slagle and Award of Merit in the context of the 1950s and 1960s and said:

> Back in my era we did not have many awards, we had the Slagle and Award of Merit. I think the greatest thrill of all, without a doubt was the Slagle, because it was only the third Slagle. I felt [it was] very treasured to have a Slagle. It was more academically oriented than say the Lindy Boggs award that was political. I thought for 10 months before I wrote it, and struggled with it. (Wiemer/Peters oral history, April 18–19, 2003, lines 4,505–4,510; 5,902–5,910)

Reflecting on her close community connections while showing me her Award of Merit, Wiemer said she was proud of it because she believed Ruth Robinson wrote the tribute. She said, "I suspect she [Robinson] did it; I don't know. It just sounded like her" (Wiemer/Peters oral history, April 18–19, 2003, line 4,523–4,526). She added:

> I never thought of myself as a leader, even though it happened. I thought of myself as a practitioner. To have Maryland OT establish an award in my name was just one of the most humbling things that could happen. It's been a very fulfilling career for me. I've never had a day's regret choosing OT. The thread throughout my career has been the marvelous women I met, the OTs and their personal strength. You make friendships that you never lose. It's just been a joy to be part of it. (Wiemer/Peters oral history, March 18–19, 2003, lines 5,950–5,953; 5,893–5,900; 6,482–6,490)

Wiemer's inner circle of friends included community insider Wilma West. Like close colleague Fidler, she received the Wilma L. West AOTA and AOTF President's Commendation in 1998. Receiving this occupational therapy lifetime achievement award in West's name is a poignant homage to their friendship. Wiemer worked for the Maryland State Department of Health from 1962 until 1980, and West worked for the Department of Health, Maternal and Child Bureau in Washington during that period. They combined their occupational therapy advocacy efforts. Like others West teamed with, Wiemer complemented West to form a powerful team. They hired rehabilitation lobbyist Russell Dean and successfully put occupational therapy on legislative agendas.

Based in Baltimore, Wiemer knew physicians and occupational therapy supporters William Rush Dunton, Jr., and Winthrop M. Phelps. Wiemer fondly remembered attending Maryland state occupational therapy meetings at the Shephard and Enoch Pratt Hospital or Johns Hopkins Hospital with Dunton and community member Robert Bing.

Wiemer first met Phelps in 1940 while doing her pediatric internship at the Children's Rehabilitation Institute or the Phelps Clinic. After being graduated-from the Philadelphia School of Occupational Therapy, she worked at the Phelps clinic from 1941–1961. Phelps was an expert and researcher, working with children who had cerebral palsy. With Phelps' encouragement and example, Wiemer began writing about her work at the Phelps Clinic. In 1947 she authored her first chapter about cerebral palsy in former teachers' Willard and Spackman's first edition (Willard & Spackman, 1947) of *The Principles of Occupational Therapy*, in 1947, and then also in Dunton and Licht's (Dunton & Licht, 1950); *Occupational Therapy Principles and Practice* in 1950. Her connection to both Willard and Spackman started in her student days. Fondly recalling her first Willard meeting and admission interview at the Philadelphia School, Wiemer said:

> I was interviewing and Helen Willard, looked up and said, 'There's a hurricane, you'd better get going.' I got on the train in Philadelphia. What should have been an hour or hour-and-a-half ride, wasn't. I left at 4:00 PM and got home about two in the morning. I was soaking wet, in my Peck and Peck suit, but I decided I wanted OT. I entered the certificate program. (Wiemer/Peters oral history, April 18–19, 2003, lines 322–342)

Wiemer found her career rewarding (Brunyate, 1954a, 1954b, 1962, 1963a, 1963b, 1964, 1966, 1967a, 1967b, 1968, 1970). She added, "I was fascinated with the practical clinical work I did, then later with the administrative work." (line 6,484). She was so invested in her career, that she almost missed out on marriage. Wiemer said:

> I got so busy with my career and interested in everything that I almost missed out on marriage. I was content, happy, and busy. I'm certainly glad I didn't miss it, but I didn't marry until my 50s. I didn't soon enough.

I say to younger OTs, don't make OT your social life as well as your professional life. My close friends were my professional friends; they're not my neighbors. (Wiemer/Peters oral history, April 18–19, 2003, lines 531–558)

Wiemer, known as Ruth Brunyate to the community, remained single until she retired at 53. She tells about marrying former hospital administrator and supervisor, Christopher Wiemer. She said:

I think, unlike the others who you interviewed, I dropped out more than the rest of them in terms of when I stopped working. My husband chased me for 12 years. I went on with my professional affairs; I was busy at all hours of the night. I was out of town and he would meet me at the airport. He was very tolerant of my professional life. So when I married, I felt I owed him all my life and time. That was October 1979. (Weimer/Peters oral history, March 18–19, 2003, lines 562–585)

Brunyate met Wiemer when he was the executive director of the Children's Rehabilitation Institute (CRI) in Baltimore. She worked under his supervision as administrative assistant and became acting director in 1957 while he was ill. CRI disbanded as the Phelps Clinic in the early 1960s, and was renamed the Kennedy Children's Center and is now part of Johns Hopkins Hospital. Dedicating her Slagle lecture to mentors Helen Willard and Christopher Weimer, Ruth Brunyate Wiemer recalled Christopher Wiemer's belief that occupational therapy professionalism was important and said:

He arrived at CRI two months before an [1955] OT conference in Houston. He said, 'When are you leaving?' I said, 'I'm not going.' When he asked why not, I said, 'I can't even get there.' He picked up the phone and called PanAm, made flight reservations and said, 'You go.' That was my first conference and Stattel's Slagle. I had been to a conference before in Washington, but we sneaked out at night and came back. Our boss wouldn't let us go. He just didn't believe in it at all. (Wiemer/Peters oral history, March 18–19, 2003, lines 1,367–1,428)

Wiemer chose a different path than her mother, who was a homemaker, mother of two, and an attorney's wife. Her mother was widowed while Wiemer was attending the Philadelphia School of Occupational Therapy. Wiemer lived with her mother during her adult life, providing financial and emotional support. Wiemer, who coped with childhood rheumatic fever that influenced her career choice, remembered her mother and said:

"I had rheumatic fever as a child, and was bedridden for most of the year. My mother managed me. I grew up in a family where you did handiwork. My mother and my aunts all did sewing, needlepoint, and knitting. I grew up doing that. I lived across the street from school, so I could see the kids go back and forth. The policeman on the corner eventually came and carried me downstairs so I could see the kids, and then carried me back when he went off duty. The experience made me interested in health. I was a young girl and I grew up watching my peers go off and do things that I couldn't. (Wiemer/Peters oral history, April 18–19, 2003, lines 292–320)

Wiemer's mother, like Yerxa's and Fidler's mothers, was unable to complete a university degree. Wiemer talked about her parents, their backgrounds, and their commitment to a college education. She stated:

Mother was born in Vineland, New Jersey. My father's father was a minister from Nova Scotia who eventually came to South Jersey. Dad moved all over. My mother lost her mother, and had to raise her five siblings. At that time she was enrolled at Goucher, and had to come home instead. After she married my father, she was embarrassed about not going to college. So he designed a college course for her and home taught her. They were fascinating, both grand people.

I grew up in the depression and my father had two of us in college at the same time. I wanted to go to OT school, but my family insisted on college first. I went to Hollins, majored in sociology. I had a rough time the first year. I was a disaster scholastically. I stuck with Hollins and graduated on the dean's list. Then I went into OT. (Wiemer/Peters oral history, April 18–19, 2003, lines 1,053–1,063; 240–253; 193–217)

Although both parents influenced Wiemer's success, she speaks about her father as her intellectual role model as well as her moral beacon. Wiemer credits her own writing skills to her father's abilities. So moved by her father's writings, Wiemer quoted from a letter he wrote her in 1935 in her Slagle lecture about clinical education. Sharing a student's perspective, she asked clinical educators to understand how difficult it can be when young students leave their families. One cannot help but think that her Slagle was autobiographical, reflecting her undergraduate time away from home as well as her own clinical internships. In the following citation, Wiemer's father explained moral character:

If he gains an appreciation of the good, which is inherent in every fellow being whatever his station in life, and a commiseration for the evil, again in every human being whatever his claim to godliness, then he will be able to secure his own personal code of behavior upon which he will operate for the rest of his days. (Brunyate, 1958, p. 198)

Wiemer received frequent letters from her father while she struggled in her early undergraduate education at Hollins College, a women's liberal arts university. This support gave her self-confidence. Being graduated on the dean's list, she succeeded beyond early academic expectations. Wiemer went on to earn her occupational therapy certificate from the University of Pennsylvania in 1940 and a Master of Education from Johns Hopkins University in 1967. She was honored with an Honorary Doctor of Letters (LHD) from Towson University in 1980. Putting her freshman struggles in context, Wiemer's father writes:

> Make the best of it, and have a good time. Don't take your work too seriously, for nobody, including yourself, will be greatly harmed by it 100 year hence. Work is important of course, but health and happiness are far more so. Life is too short to forgo any real pleasure you can get out of it. (Wiemer/Peters oral history, April 18–19, 2003, lines 3,515–3,522)

Weimer's father died unexpectedly in 1939 when she, at age 23, was enrolled at the Philadelphia School. Mentor and community old guard, Willard, was very understanding during this difficult period in Wiemer's life. Losing her father was life-changing in many ways. Talking about him, Wiemer shared that he was an attorney who helped the underdog, and showed me newspaper clippings in her private papers from cases stating, "Heavyweight Boxer Ernie Shaft III Featured in New York Match with Primo Carnera." (line 3,561) Weimer recalled her formative years visiting her father's Newark, New Jersey office which introduced her to the work world. She stated:

> I remember I used to go down to his office when his secretary was on vacation, and answer the phones, and peck away at the typewriter. He'd take me to lunch. We walked down Broad Street towards Schrafft's. My father took his walking stick. (Wiemer/Peters oral history, April 18–19, 2003, lines 1,038–1,047)

The death of Wiemer's father also created a situation where she stayed longer at the Philadelphia School, and spent more time with Willard and Spackman as a result. This additional time together cemented their lifelong relationship. Wiemer explained:

> I was with them longer than usual because of my father's death. They shifted my clinicals around. Pediatrics first, and then I was back with Claire for phys dys [physical dysfunction] when this happened. I stayed in Philadelphia so I could get home to my mother on weekends and help give her support through it all. So Helen and Claire restructured that to keep me in Philadelphia. I saw them constantly. It helped me see the inner workings of AOTA sooner than I would have, through them. (Wiemer/Peters oral history, April 18–19, 2003, lines 383–419)

Wiemer cherished her relationship with Willard, who mentored and introduced her to the community. Honoring Willard, Wiemer saved a November 3, 1961, Western Union telegram from Lucy Blair on behalf of the American Physical Therapy Association congratulating AOTA immediate past President Willard for a successful conference marking the "growth and development of the profession" (Wiemer, private papers, 1961). Willard handed her presidency over to newly-elected Wilma West in Detroit at that conference, representing another Wiemer connection.

Just days after that telegram, Wiemer as first vice president elect during West's presidency, introduced the community of therapists who were seated at the head banquet table at the Detroit conference table on November 7, 1961. The evening banquet was AOTA's formal black-tie event that followed the Slagle lecture, and gave a glimpse of the association's leaders: Lyla Spelbring, president of the Michigan Occupational Therapy Association, and the conference co-chair; Marjorie Fish, the AOTA executive director, "who stands alone for her unique ability to relate to other health services;" Helen Willard, "immediate past president, known to us through long service on the board;" Ruth Robinson, "her predecessor was elder statesman to Miss Willard's Junior statesman;" Clare S. Spackman, president of the World Federation of Occupational Therapists; Myra McDaniel, second vice president, serving with the Army Medical Services at Walter Reed Hospital and commended for writing about Army history; Margaret Gleave, treasurer and permanent conference chairperson who "comes in and out of the association through the years and just when done, we call again;" Ethel Huebner, speaker of the House of Delegates, "we know her for her precision attention to detail and skill;" and Barbara Jewett, local conference co-chair. That evening, Wiemer also recognized Michigan's occupational therapy "history makers, Lyla Spelbring and Marion Spear," (AOTA 1961 Banquet Program, Sheraton Hotel, Detroit, Michigan, November 7, 1961, Wiemer, private notes).[23] Spelbring, an AOTA and AOTF leader, was a close colleague of community members Cromwell and Welles. Spear was community member Llorens' academic program director and mentor at Wayne State University.

Known as a clinician, administrator, and leader, Wiemer established herself at the Children's Rehabilitation Institute (1941–1961), Milwaukee–Downer College (1961), and served at the Maryland State Department of Health, renamed the Department of Health and Mental Hygiene (1962–1980). Politically, she helped establish and chair AOTA's Legislative Affairs Committee between 1968 and 1973. Marion Crampton remembers no one else as more capable to lead that committee than Wiemer. The Legislative Affairs Committee later expanded to the Government Affairs division of AOTA. Somewhat conservative and different in style from Florence Cromwell who followed her as AOTA president, Weimer understood Washington, DC, in the 1960s and 1970s and occupational therapy's inner circles.

Florence Cromwell

Florence Cromwell was a political mover and an AOTA Award of Merit recipient in 1974. In 1999 she received a lifetime achievement award, and the AOTA and AOTF President's Commendation, which was named after Wilma West (AOTA, 1975). In her two terms as AOTA's president, immediately following Wiemer in 1967–1970, and 1970–1973, she uprooted the northeastern AOTA presidential tradition. Taking office as a California-based therapist, she activated a grass roots effort at the state level throughout the country. This came from her state-level involvement in the Occupational Therapy Association of California (OTAC) since 1949 and continues today. For example, in her first years as a therapist, she was president of the then Southern California Occupational Therapy Association from 1950 to 1951.

Cromwell was a leader with a clear vision. She retired in 1988, and her career spanned 25 years of working in physical rehabilitation and community-based, work-oriented program administration, like the Los Angeles Job Corps. Earning a second baccalaureate degree, a Bachelor of Science in Occupational Therapy from Washington University in 1949, and a Master of Arts in Occupational Therapy from the University of Southern California in 1952, she came into the community of therapists with a combination of the right schooling and knowing the right people. Yerxa remembered her student internship under Cromwell, and identified her as instilling a sense of professionalism. Exploring new roles for occupational therapy, Cromwell was a researcher for the United Cerebral Palsy Association of Los Angeles between 1956 and 1960. She was also the occupational therapy coordinator in the Division of Research and Training in Rehabilitation at the University of Southern California's School of Medicine from 1968 to 1970, and the acting chair of occupational therapy at the University of Southern California from 1974 to 1976. Reflecting on a career in occupational therapy, Cromwell stated:

> I can't imagine having had a career in anything that would have given me both the opportunity and the richness of experience that I have had. I've been lucky, and I got to know the right people at the right times. The decisions about where I worked and what I did were fortuitous. The professionalization that occurred started while I was in school. I got to meet all the bigwigs that we read about and heard about while a student. Everybody knew everybody; they were all great buddies. (Cromwell/Peters oral history, April 28–29, 2005, lines 7,890–7,917)

Cromwell, called Crum by her life partner for more than 50 years, Carlotta Welles, and other therapists, explained her informal name, illustrating community connections and insider intimacies.She explained, "Carlotta's sister named me Crum, short for Crumbly. To her parents and everybody, and a lot of the OTs, I'm Crum" (Cromwell/Peters oral history, April 28–29, 2003, lines 8,743–8,749).

Although she has been a Los Angeles, California-based occupational therapist since 1949, she was born in Chester, Pennsylvania. Cromwell's father worked for Baldwin Locomotive as a design engineer before relocating the family to New Jersey and Ohio during the depression years. The Cromwell name is linked to the eastern railroad industry. About this she stated, "My parents were from Baltimore, and my father's family was in the railroad industry as design engineers for generations. The A.J. Cromwell Museum in Baltimore is my father's great grandfather" (Cromwell/Peters oral history, April 28–29, 2003, lines 186–194). Like others in the community, Cromwell's father thought it was important for her to have a practical college education. She explains:

> When the time came to go to school, no one had gone to college. My mother hadn't. My father and his brother had college degrees. Father went to Hopkins. Dad said, 'We'll manage it somehow, but be sure to choose something where you can get a job.' (Cromwell/Peters oral history, April 28–29, 2003, lines 252–255, 203–211)

Cromwell chose teaching although she did not pursue the career because she was sidetracked by World War II. Shewas graduated from Miami University in Ohio in 1943 with a Bachelor of Science degree in Elementary and Secondary Education. Showing early leadership skills at Miami University that continued to her AOTA presidency, she was the president of the Kappa Kappa Gamma (Delta Lambda) social fraternity in 1942 and 1943 at Miami University. She also was a member of the Mortar Board, a senior women's honorary, in 1942. Speaking about her undergraduate college affiliations she remembered:

> I was a Mortar Board member, which is a senior women's honor that was very select. My sorority was colonized (incorporated) in my freshman year, and I couldn't afford it. By the next year my sisters were both working and said they would help me, so my sophomore and junior year I was pledge chairman. By my senior year I was president. Having done those things, I was president of my OT class. There were only nine of us in the class, three of us veterans. (Cromwell/Peters oral history, April 28–29, 2003, lines 7,953–7,992; 8,009–8,014)

Following her graduation, Cromwell enlisted and remembered her military experience as a woman officer. She stated:

> I graduated in elementary education in 1943 when the war and the WAVES [Women Accepted for Volunteer Emergency Service] started.

I was a WAVE officer stationed in Washington [DC] in an administrative role; no differences between men and women in the Navy hierarchy. The head of the WAVES was Mildred MacAfee, who was the president of Wellesley College. She robbed all the Ivy League schools of top women to staff the WAVES organization. Classes commenced at Smith College in Massachusetts for officers. They were recruiting college and professional women with a high level of professionalism. The GI Bill made my graduate education possible in 1946. Those war years provided the important beginning to my professional life in occupational therapy. (Cromwell/ Peters oral history, April 28–29, 2003, lines 277–288; 2,462–2,475; 318–322; 335; 355; 2,432–2,434; 2,469–2,475. U.S. Navy WAVES, Cromwell unpublished speech, January 2001)

Seeking another career after serving in the United States Naval Reserve from 1943 until 1946, Cromwell learned about occupational therapy from close family friends she identified as Aunt Lar and Uncle Lee. Their youngest daughter, Ann, had just been graduated from the Philadelphia School of Occupational Therapy, and Cromwell thought that was a "reasonable thing to do," (line 375). While visiting her sister in St. Louis, she went to Washington University, inquiring about the occupational therapy program. She stated, "Washington University was literally dying for students because of the war. They enrolled me instantly. They were charmed to get three veterans who could pay full tuition." (Cromwell/Peters, oral history, April 28–29, 2003, lines 388–395)

Cromwell's occupational therapy internships influenced her career path and her entrance to the community of therapists. Remembering her psychiatric internship at the Veterans Administration Hospital in Lawrence, Kansas in 1947 reminded her of the war years and the gender biases women therapy interns faced. This experience along with others spurred Cromwell's quest for professionalism. She stated:

It was very traumatic personally, because I had never been around anybody who had mental illness before. These were all our contemporaries. I had been in the war, but here were all these ex-soldiers, -marines, and -navy people so sick. Because we were all women students in most disciplines, we had to be at the swimming pool, do the dances and everything. (Cromwell/Peters oral history, April 28–29, 2003, lines 7,810–7,832)

Her internship was at Los Angeles County General Hospital under Carlotta Welles' supervision. This led to her first staff therapist position in 1949 which lasted until 1953. Cromwell, showing great talent, became Occupational Therapy Department Chief Welles' assistant. A strong individual, Cromwell was not one to stay in Welles' shadow, but rather quickly became an equal. Welles, 15 years Cromwell's senior, and a Boston School graduate,

along with classmate West, bridged occupational therapy leadership generations, dating back to AOTA President Kahmann who served from 1947 until
1952. Welles, an active AOTA committee member, knew many established
therapists and influential people whom Cromwell met early in her career.
Thus Cromwell achieved her community insider status.

With community support, Cromwell guided and created a stronger,
more independent AOTA during her presidency (Cromwell, 1968a, 1968b,
1968c, 1968d, 1968e, 1969a, 1969b, 1969c, 1969d, 1969e, 1970a, 1970b,
1970c, 1972d, 1973a). Changes in her two terms included relocating the
national headquarters from New York to Washington, DC, and expanding
AOTA's political base. For example, Cromwell participated in the newly
formed Coalition of Independent Health Professions in 1969 until 1974.
She chaired the group of multidisciplined health care professions in 1974.
Cromwell described this group that later dissolved and stated:

> I was chairman of the Coalition of Independent Health Professions. It
> started about 1970 or '71. The first chairman was the executive director of
> speech and hearing. Everybody was beginning to recognize that you had
> to be in Washington, DC, for political clout. We had nursing, osteopaths,
> social workers, podiatrists, PT, and OT. The big wheels were in it, and
> the limitation was we never could come to an agreement for any position
> papers that would satisfy the whole membership. It was the time of
> Medicare. (Cromwell/Peters oral history, April 28–29, 2003, lines
> 1,331–1,355)

Recalling the time when the Medicare Bill was on Washington's legislative
docket, Cromwell remembered some of her Health, Education, and Welfare
dealings that continued from Wiemer's AOTA presidency. She stated:

> The regulations were being ground out of HEW at that time. We had a leg
> up because we had Willie (West). She was in a powerful position. And
> Marge Fish had been there before her. That was when we had another
> woman who we couldn't bear, I don't want to use her name, but she
> was anything but helpful to us. We were undercut in many ways. I remem-
> ber a meeting in Bethesda at some funky little motel where the OTs were
> deciding about this (Medicare). Gail (Fidler) was fuming, and I was fum-
> ing, not knowing how to solve it. We had Russ (lobbyist Russell Dean). He
> was our voice in Washington. It was only after Leo (Fanning) got in office
> that we began to have a Government Affairs person. (Cromwell/Peters
> oral history, April 28–29, 2003, lines 6,498–6,537, 1,394–1,432)

Another Cromwell concern for an independent profession related to
occupational therapy setting its own educational standards (Cromwell
1970a; Cromwell & Kielhofner, 1976). Traditionally, occupational therapy
educational standards functioned under the auspices of the American Medical
Association. Cromwell, viewing the profession's dilemmas on a broader level,

thought the problem was larger. Adding to the mix, states started licensing occupational therapy. Cromwell remembered:

> With the coming of licensure has been the weakening of AOTA. They (therapists) don't look to us for standards and the definition of what the profession should be. I was on accreditation for 7 years in the late 70 s. When more states got licensed they thought, 'Well we just have to meet whatever their states said.' I felt very strongly that we had to loudly pronounce that we're the ones to set the standards for the field, for education, for certification and for the things that make a good product, and a good therapist with ethical standards. Other people would have said we should have gone with the flow, go with what the feds were doing, big government is better. I think people were thinking the government is going to take over the health business, you better be with that team. I believed strongly in the principles of our founders. If we were under the control of somebody else who dictated what we should have in our course work, what would that mean? (Cromwell/Peters oral history, April 28–29, 2005, lines 1,442–1,467; 4,831–4,836; 8,176–8,191)

Cromwell remained a strong and thoughtful spokesperson for occupational therapy's uniqueness and betterment. Given an impressive record for change, I asked her if there were any goals that she had not achieved. Her response summarized her keen career actions and her humility. She said:

> You don't know if you will always grab every opportunity that would have been. Possibly I wasn't terribly courageous. I needed to break new ground. I guess we just try to do what seemed right at the time according to the trends and decide what was demanded. (Cromwell/Peters oral history, April 28–29, 2003, lines 8,305–8,313)

If Cromwell represents a 1970s political mover, the last political community member Elnora Gilfoyle, shaped 1980s AOTA during her presidency. Like other leaders, her influence began years before, in the 1960s and 1970s.

Elnora M. Gilfoyle

My first impression upon meeting Elnora Gilfoyle at her suburban home not far from Estes Park, Colorado, was how her comfort with people, her hearty laugh, and gusto dwarfed her six-foot height. Elnora M. Gilfoyle shaped occupational therapy politically when she was AOTA's president between 1986 and 1989 (Gilfoyle, 1986a, 1986b, 1986c, 1987a, 1987b, 1987c, 1988), and intellectually, when she received the Eleanor Clarke Slagle lectureship in 1984, and the Award of Merit in 1991. Contributing to occupational therapy's literature, Gilfoyle and (Ann) Grady (1971, 1978) and Gilfoyle, Grady, and Moore (1981) in *Children Adapt* presents a developmental theory of spatiotemporal adaptation. The spatiotemporal adaptation theory explains how a child's development results from a child's interaction with his or her world. Maturation is an ongoing and continuous adaptation or spiraling process. According to the authors, maturation for children with disabilities is dependent upon subcortical learning and environmental modifications facilitated by the therapist.

Gilfoyle began her career in Denver, Colorado in 1956, working as an occupational therapist in adult and pediatric rehabilitation at two hospitals, including the now renowned Craig Rehabilitation Hospital. In the early 1960s she established herself in pediatric occupational therapy rehabilitation and research at The Denver Children's Hospital and the John F. Kennedy Child Development Center prior to starting as a faculty member at Colorado State University in the 1980s, and advancing to an Associate Dean in 1988. (AOTA, 1988). Gilfoyle, a retired provost and academic vice president of Colorado State University (1991–1995), received an Honarary Doctorate of Science, from that same university in 1981. Gilfoyle was the first occupational therapist to receive an honorary Doctor of Science degree, a year after Wiemer's Honorary Doctor of Humane Letters (AOTA, 1981, p. 1). Committed to Colorado State University and occupational therapy, a politically experienced Gilfoyle spoke about how she strategized to keep a floundering occupational therapy program alive in the 1980s at Colorado State University. She stated:

> I was real political, I knew what needed to be done. We needed an [occupational therapy] identity. How do you get an identity? Get out there and market yourself with articles in the paper and going to faculty meetings. You get people involved in the university; you get a building named after yourself. You apply for all the honors that you could possibly get at the university to get the recognition that you need. (Gilfoyle/Peters oral history, February 10–11, 2003, lines 2,826–2,836)

As a community insider, Gilfoyle suggested that her Colorado Occupational Therapy Association involvement was one of her stepping stones to national level leadership. From her earliest introduction, like others in the community, Gilfoyle, who was known as Ellie to her peers, was linked to Wilma West. Remembering her community introductions and AOTA political involvement, Gilfoyle stated:

> We were so small it was easy to be part of the inner core because there just weren't that many people. I had a firm belief in the strength of an association, in the strength of a community. I was real active in the Colorado OT Association. Being chair of that [Denver AOTA] conference put me into AOTA. I ran for secretary of AOTA, that was my real entry. I don't think anybody knew me. I was elected secretary and Jerry Johnson was president at the time.[24] (Gilfoyle/Peters oral history, February 10–11, 2003, lines 951–966)

Gilfoyle described her relationship with another community member and close colleague, Ann Grady, as a sisterhood. Grady, a more recent AOTA president and Eleanor Clarke Slagle recipient, had her own community entrance via her mentor, Mary Fiorentino.[25] Putting the Gilfoyle and Grady team on the community insider's radar, Gilfoyle remembered a West-financed 1970s symposium that led to the publishing of *Children Adapt* (Gilfoyle, Grady, & Moore, 1981). Sensorimotor adaptation, the basis of the book, led to more than 150 workshops and 50 professional papers on the subject (AOTA, 1986). In the community of therapists, West's symposia were vehicles for inner circle networking and introducing occupational therapy's new talent. Gilfoyle remembered her first symposium and stated:

> We [Gilfoyle and Grady] were a team unto ourselves, other than Jean Ayres. We'd talk to her, but not so much about publishing. We were really a team. What did we know about writing, nothing. But we did it. It [*Children Adapt*] came out of the Boston Symposium. It was like we were on stage and going to perform. We had this flannel board. I talked and the flannel board fell down in front of Jean Ayres, Anne Henderson, Willie West and Jo [Josephine] Moore. It was a three-ring circus. We were trying to impress people. We didn't have to do that. (Gilfoyle/Peters oral history, February 10–11, 2003, lines 1,562–1,586)

Modeling herself after strong independent community members, Gilfoyle started her quest to help empower women occupational therapists. Comfortable wearing feminist shoes while being a practitioner, educator, administrator, or consultant, she balanced the life roles of career woman, wife, mother, daughter, and sister. The following quotation illustrates Gilfoyle's feminist convictions:

> I never felt that I wasn't in charge of myself, or that I had to succumb. A lot was feeling confident enough in myself and understanding what was. In our society it is a male hierarchy, because it's primarily the men who have been out there. I think Rosie the Riveter had a lot more to do with the evolution of women than NOW [National Organization of Women]. I think NOW pulled us back a little bit. It's the 'I Can Do' that is going to get us somewhere. (Gilfoyle/Peters oral history, February 10–11, 2003, line 1,857–1,870)

As a self-proclaimed realist, Gilfoyle grappled with gender barriers as a student like other young women in the 1950s with limited study options. These early experiences stirred her desire to change an unfair status quo. She stated:

> I didn't really know what I wanted to go into; interior designer, science teacher or social worker like my sister. That was the 50 s. That was in the

days that all I really wanted to do was get married and have a family. Anything I wanted to major in as a woman was primarily through home economics. I got Cs and Ds because I didn't shine the chrome or clean the cooking tools. I thought I can't believe this is going on in life. They discouraged woman from doing anything in sciences. I didn't like that. I just thought that's really closing the door. (Gilfoyle/Peters oral history, February 10–11, 2003, lines 16–43)

Gilfoyle learned that 1950s female stereotypes prevailed in occupational therapy as well as home economics. Consistent with other community members' reports, occupational therapy enrollment numbers were small in the 1950s. Remembering her occupational therapy entrance interview at the State University of Iowa in Iowa City, after transferring from a home economics major at Iowa State University in Ames, a disappointed Gilfoyle stated:

In order to get into OT, I had to have an interview and thought, 'This is really prestigious.' All they talked about was that I was very tall, and that I made all my clothes, so we talked about sewing. I left thinking, 'This is worse than Iowa State.' I was so disappointed. They were screaming for kids to major and there was no competition. I was in a class of seven. (Gilfoyle/Peters oral history, February 10–11, 2003, lines 87–96)

Similar to other community members, Gilfoyle credits her self-esteem to her father through the life lessons he taught her. In paying homage to her father, she said she cherishes a traditional German wood cabinet in her home that her father made. She explained that he treated his daughters as equals with his son and thought women could hold their weight in the work force. Gilfoyle, an Iowa native, spoke about her early family years that helped define her beliefs and career path. She stated:

I was the youngest of four siblings in a German family with a strong work ethic. We were very poor but didn't know it. I wasn't a depression baby; I was at the end of that. My father was an astounding man, never graduated from high school, but a sheer genius. He developed a machine lathe tool.

I never felt that work was not for women. I worked in a machine shop with my brother and my sisters. Working in the machine shop gave me practical experience that I used with orthotics and prosthetics. I never felt any stigma being a woman. I told my father I think I want to be an artist. He said, 'No, I'm sending you to school to prepare for a career.' I decided to become an OT. Had it been ten years later, I would have majored in engineering, but that wasn't open to me as a woman. I never thought about going into medicine.

My father said, 'One thing I want you to remember in life. You can go as far as you want in life. You can do anything you want as long as you don't care who gets the credit.' You do things for the betterment of others. That's the way he lived, and that's the way we all lived. (Gilfoyle/Peters oral history, February 10–11, 2003, lines 630–684; 690–704; 717–720)

Continuing to challenge traditional female role hurdles, Gilfoyle believed "you can be a very happy and successful wife, mother, and career person," (line 3,189). She acknowledges that much of her career and personal support came from husband of 50 years, Gene, and son Sean. As a mother, Gilfoyle remembered when a journalist interviewed her son about his reaction to his mother's provost position at Colorado State University. She stated:

> Because I was the first woman provost at Colorado, some magazine writers interviewed Sean, asking him what it was like having a powerful businesswoman who was an excellent manager as a mother. He looked at them and said, 'At home my mother is not a manager, she's my mother.' I just thought, 'God, isn't that wonderful. That's what he saw.' (Gilfoyle/Peters oral history, February 10–11, 2003, lines 2,981–3,001)

Seeking career and leisure balance, Gilfoyle combined her work and social life. She recalled that occupational and physical therapists at Denver General Hospital, where she first worked built a work and social community. She said:

> Denver General was a little community. Our friendships were the people with whom I worked. We socialized together; it was sort of a life. I was married, most everyone was. Gene liked the people I worked with, so he just came along. He was my best friend and loved what was going on. I lived my OT values. I believed in the importance of recreation and leisure time. We were able to balance it in this community. On weekends we never talked about work, but we were there together. (Gilfoyle/Peters oral history, February 10–11, 2003, lines 539–575)

Combining work and play paralleled the occupational therapy community culture. Gillette described how Gilfoyle identified a pristine retreat location during her AOTA presidency when AOTF sponsored occupational therapy research seminars. Gillette stated:

> We tried to build research teams that related to practice. For the $10,000 that we had to offer them, we would take four teams at a time and take them off to the mountains. We went to this gorgeous place that Ellie Gilfoyle recommended at 9,400 feet elevation at Roosevelt National Forest. Perfectly beautiful, exactly the kind of retreat to learn in, to do research, but still have beauty around you. (Gillette/Peters interview, January 29, 2003, lines 1,560–1,574)

A continuous thread in Gilfoyle's professional life was her willingness to explore opportunities. Gilfoyle, quoted in an occupational therapy newspaper, stated, "I am fortunate to have been in situations that have afforded rich opportunities for my professional growth and development. My career has evolved from clinical practice through management to professional education and research" (Occupational Therapy News, May 1986, p. 1).

Her quest was advantageous because she gained occupational therapy research funding from 1968 to 1991 totaling $2,148,000 from agencies like the United States Public Health Services, the United States Department of Education, Maternal and Child Health Services, the United States Department of Health and Human Services, and the Colorado Department of Education. A research advocate, Gilfoyle worked closely with AOTA and AOTF, forming research partnerships. Creative Partnership, a theme in her 1987 presidential address in April at the 67th annual AOTA meeting in Indianapolis, became Gilfoyle's (1987b) term for occupational therapy's partnerships as linkages for preserving caring and other traditional values in an entrepreneurial world. She prioritized the blending of science and art to promote a better quality of life for those served by occupational therapists. She explained:

> We [AOTA] were really about promoting a creative partnership with the foundation and promoting research. One of the things that happened is we passed a measure in the Representative Assembly to provide 2% of membership dues to the Foundation. I thought every therapist should contribute to the promotion of the profession and the foundation. The foundation is created to promote the profession through research and education. (Gilfoyle/Peters oral history, February 10–11, 2003, lines 2,316–2,325)

Still active, Gilfoyle currently facilitates corporate leadership seminars for women that echo her occupational therapy feminist themes. Froehlich (1992) identified Gilfoyle's occupational therapy theme as self-esteem, modeling a belief that good leaders care for themselves and their constituencies. Seeing herself as a can-do woman, Gilfoyle summarized her beliefs and said:

> I think I model hope and opportunities. It's amazing when I think I became a provost. It was amazing when I became a dean. I was the first one [in occupational therapy], but now we have other deans like Chuck [Christiansen] and Nancy Talbot. Being an occupational therapist provided a foundation, a core for so many different areas. There is hope and possibilities for each of us. I hope that someday people will say, 'Oh yes, she did know that.' (Gilfoyle/Peters oral history, February 10–11, 2003, lines 3,176–3,187)

Political movers Ruth Brunyate Wiemer, Florence Cromwell, and Elnora Gilfoyle represented the 1950s, 1960s, and 1970s community of therapists. They all had leadership skills and were AOTA presidents. Wiemer, remaining single for most of her work life, excelled as a bureaucrat; Cromwell, Carlotta Welles' life partner, worked as a community-based therapist and educator; and Gilfoyle, married with a son, worked as an academic administrator. Each redefined occupational therapy. What was common to them was their belief in occupational therapy's worth, and their talent for finding and developing opportunities.

The following section introduces the occupational therapy sustainers. These therapists worked to keep a strong occupational therapy infrastructure through their intellectual pursuits, financial and work contributions. There are two sustainer categories, reflecting different time frames: old guard sustainers, Boston and Philadelphia school graduates who excelled in the 1950s and 1960s and the new-guard sustainers who represented a changing occupational therapy in the 1960s and 1970s.

Old and New Guard Sustainers

Alphabetically presented, Marion Crampton, Florence Stattel, and Carlotta Welles were occupational therapy's old guard sustainers. Contemporaries, Crampton and Welles were graduated from the Boston School, while Stattel was graduated from the Philadelphia School. Aside from their common East Coast professional occupational therapy education, these women differed in career paths and private lives. Although as a group there are some parallels, like family upbringing, and their career-long belief in occupational therapy.

New guard sustainers Robert K. Bing and Lela A. Llorens represented occupational therapy's firsts. Bing, a former academic dean and occupational therapy historian, was the first and only male occupational therapist elected AOTA president. Llorens, a former academic vice president, and scholar, was the first and only African American woman to receive the Eleanor Clarke Slagle lectureship. Bing and Llorens broke new ground and created new occupational therapy infrastructures for future generations.

Like the theorists and futurists, political movers, old- and new-guard sustainers can be linked to Wilma West. These five therapists knew West as a classmate, friend, mentor, or professional supporter.

Marion W. Crampton

Marion Wright Crampton remembered wearing the Boston School's blue occupational therapy student uniform with white starched collar and cuffs, required in 1935. Crampton stated that occupational therapy graduates wore all white uniforms. She conformed to student protocol, unlike her friend Gail Fidler who rarely wore her Philadelphia School green uniform with the required starched white collar and cuffs. Crampton, a 1935 Wellesley College graduate and Spanish major prior to her occupational therapy education, adhered to the Boston school's protocol. Unassuming and gracious, she had a quiet reserve and humbleness about her occupational therapy contributions that were laced with her quick, dry wit. A community of therapists insider, Crampton exemplified the type of young woman occupational therapy educational program directors recruited in the 1930s. She was well-educated, cultured, and seeking adventurous new experiences.

Raised in a white, upper-middle class family, she never married. Discreet about her socioeconomic background, she shared, "In the summer we were always in the Vineyard (referring to the Cape Cod resort area, Martha's Vineyard), (line 295). As did community member Wiemer, she enjoyed her career development and dedicated herself to her family responsibilities. She spoke about how her family background guided her career selection. Influenced by her father, like other community members, Crampton's long-standing New England heritage echoed the values of a comfortable middle class, stating:

> Dennis Crampton came to this country from Ireland and married a New Englander who was English, Scotch and Irish. My father was born in Concord [Massachusetts], then moved to California and Vermont. His mother traveled and had a home in Woodstock, Vermont. That was for summer, spring, and fall. They would stay at an apartment in Brookline in the winter, or in Arizona. (Crampton/Peters oral history, March 1, 2003, lines 34–66, 2,832–2,848)

Crampton lives alone in a stately Boston architect-designed three-story Arlington, Massachusetts home, the same family house that she has lived in since 1914. As befitting an occupational therapist trained in the arts and crafts movement, there are handcrafted items that she has made in the house, including some wood sculpture. Crampton spoke about learning woodcarving when she worked as the director of occcupational therapy at Queens Hospital in Honolulu, Hawaii from 1940–1941, leaving just prior to the Pearl Harbor attack. She recalled:

> I took up wood carving. The teacher was at the Honolulu Academy or art museum. He learned how to carve in Switzerland. He could see wood, and see the form in it. We had gotten the wood from Duke Kahanamoku, the Olympic swimmer who was working in corrections.[26] I made a head sculpture and brought it back. I have it in my bedroom upstairs. (Crampton/Peters oral history, March 1, 2003, lines 746–765)

Crampton studied occupational therapy when science, arts, and crafts were combined, recalling:

> We had a lot of courses I already had at Wellesley: the anatomy and physiology. But we had all the craft courses too. (Crampton/Peters oral history, March 1, 2003, lines 120–124)

Crampton showed me her BSOT rush stool that she made nearly 70 years before. Crampton's alumni ties remain active. Recently she was the guest of honor at a celebration marking BSOT's history. Current chair Sharon L. Schwartzberg said, "The history of BSOT largely remains unwritten. The history informs us about the evolution of a profession and the role of gender and other sociopolitical concerns that shape health care." Graduates like Crampton, Reilly, Welles, and West contributed much to the profession (BSOT, 2004, pp. 2–3).

Crampton found out about occupational therapy through a family physician and explained:

> I didn't know what I wanted to do when I was a senior in college. I thought about being a translator, but thought it would mean going to a foreign country and living with a family. I was talking to our family doctor and he said, what do you like to do? I said I liked people and I like to do things with my hands. I went to the career department at Wellesley and they told me about the Boston School of Occupational Therapy. (Crampton/Peters oral history, March 1, 2003, lines 6–17, 93–95)

Both Crampton and Stattel, who are contemporaries and old guard sustainers, came to occupational therapy wanting to help people and use their hands. They did not discuss wanting to be scientists when they initially studied occupational therapy. Rather, Crampton discussed her interest in activities. An accomplished swimmer and skilled at playing various musical instruments, she spoke about activity-based treatment in psychiatry. Working at Metropolitan State Hospital, in Waltham, Massachusetts from 1941 until 1952, she facilitated a cooking group, an exercise program, and a patient orchestra (Crampton, 1950). Crampton remembered:

> I stayed at Met State until 1953. I had an orchestra, and we played for dances every Monday night. And plays—I remember one of the plays. My sister came with her husband. One patient was a dentist who was giving my brother-in-law quite a line and my brother-in-law didn't know he was a patient. I enjoyed working with the mentally ill. (Crampton/Peters oral history, March 1, 2003, lines 863–870)

Writing about the orchestra, Crampton (1946) in an article titled "Musical Magic" stated that doctors and therapists thought mental health patients' musical interests could deepen if they worked toward some goal, thus illustrating how treatment was mutually determined by physicians and therapists in the late 1940s, and this approach carried into the 1950s. This may have implied that diversion, rather than a theoretical rationale, was the basis for treatment.

In 1952 Crampton began her 22-year position at the Massachusetts Department of Mental Health as supervisor of occupational therapy services in all of the Massachusetts state mental health hospitals. She developed curriculum to train occupational therapy assistants (Crampton, 1969; Crampton & Anderegg, 1961). Crampton wrote and received a Health

Education Welfare (HEW) training grant (No. 543-T-69, Rehabilitation Services Administration) for Massachusetts state hospital mental health aides studying to be certified occupational therapy assistants. Hiring community member and theorist Anne Mosey, as a consultant and educator, the project curriculum included a module about occupational therapy theoretical frames of reference. Expanding her work to a national level, Crampton (1961, 1967b, 1969) promoted the role of Certified Occupational Therapy Assistant (COTA) through publication and presentations. Occupational therapists throughout the country had varying responses to this effort. Cromwell and Welles, in their oral history, reported that California occupational therapists feared that COTAs would take their jobs. Crampton remembered former AOTA president Ruth Robinson being supportive because of her military experience. In contrast, Helen Willard did not want to see this new professional stratification occur. Crampton said: "Ruth Robinson had problems in the Army, and they had some kind of a program" (line 986). Related, this effort to the occupational therapy personnel shortage, Crampton chaired AOTA's personnel and finance committees from 1974 until 1976. In these positions she monitored occupational therapy's job descriptions and salary ranges. Keeping an eye on national trends, she also saw a new occupational therapy professionalism grow related to manpower demands.

Crampton received AOTA's Award of Merit in 1972 during Cromwell's presidency for her "creative imagination and persistent search for knowledge...and the acquired sophistication born of experience." Remaining understated about this honor, Crampton stated that she didn't know if she contributed enough. In her 50-year career, Crampton, with colleagues Gail Fidler and Elizabeth (Betty) Ridgway, promoted mental health practice on a national level.

Retiring in 1984 from her post as the supervisor of occupational therapy, Massachusetts Department of Mental Health, Crampton was an old guard community insider. An occupational therapist since 1937, known as Crampy by her friends, she spoke about her community sisterhood and friends Fidler and native Bostonians Ruth Robinson and Alice Jantzen; Florence Cromwell and Carlotta Welles, fellow Wellesley graduate and AOTA professional education staff member Virginia Kilburn; and AOTA certified occupational therapy assistant education committee members Mildred Schwagmeyer; and partners Naida Ackley and Ethel (Queenie) Huebner. Fidler talked about her extended stays with Crampton, stating:

> Marion Crampton, you look at who and what she was; she was absolutely wonderful, very much a colleague. I went up there regularly without my husband and did summer sessions at BU every May. Marion and I used to go to the Cape.
>
> She became a second mother to my kids, extended family. We took our son Eric on an airplane to Boston to Marion Crampton's house and

wheeled him into Boston Children's Hospital. He was in a full body cast and for 6 to 8 months he stayed with Marion. They became very, very good friends. Then our daughter Donnie [Dagny] went to school in Boston, and spent weekends at Marion's. It was absolutely wonderful. (Fidler/Peters oral history, March 6–7, 2003, lines 5,775–5,859)

As an occupational therapy leader, Crampton volunteered many hours for AOTA and a beginning AOTF (Crampton & MacDonald, 1973). Community members Fidler, Cromwell, Wiemer, and Bing agreed that Marion was the person to get a job done for the organization. Serving on AOTA's Board of Management in the 1960s, and as AOTF's inaugural secretary in 1965, Crampton received AOTF's 1981 Certificate of Appreciation. According to Wilma West, as AOTF's president, presenting the award at AOTA's conference in San Antonio, Texas, Crampton had an "unbroken record of service as an officer over 15 years during which this (AOTF, 1982) young organization developed, (p. 195). West continued:

> Her commitment to the profession has been expressed concurrently though responsibility carried out in behalf of both association and foundation. She assumed an unusual responsibility for recording not only our official actions, but also the rationale behind them. Of greatest import to the healthy status of relationships between association and foundation has been Marion's leading role in modeling the prototype for today's official liaison between respective boards. (AOTF, 1982, p. 195)

Crampton's handwritten minutes described the foundation's mission to promote occupational therapy knowledge, scientific research, and education. What was more interesting in viewing original documents was Crampton's habit of writing two sets of minutes, one official and the other with personal notes on margins that included unofficial conversation or thoughts. For example, Crampton's marginal notes highlighted the view that there was no real delineation between AOTA and AOTF when the foundation was formed (Crampton, personal papers, 1965). This is supported by the fact that AOTA board members automatically became AOTF founding board members. Hence, Crampton officially became AOTF's first secretary.

Crampton shared her perspective about being an occupational therapist, questioning whether there is something characteristic about those who enter the profession or if occupational therapy gives those who choose it a new direction. Crampton stated "I'm not sorry I became an OT. I'm glad to see the direction OT is going. I don't know if it's a part of me or if what I am doing is because of OT." (Crampton/Peters oral history, March 1, 2003, lines 2,778–2,786)

Marion Crampton, working closely with occupational therapy leaders and community members Fidler, Ridgway, Robinson, Wiemer, and West, helped sustain the infrastructure for the developing occupational therapy field. The next therapist who contributed substantially to occupational therapy's professionalization is New Yorker Florence Stattel.

Florence Stattel

Jacqueline Goldberg, a retired switchboard operator who knew Florence Stattel in the 1950s as an occupational therapist at Kessler Rehabilitation Institute in New Jersey, wrote:

> In September 1948 at the age of twenty, while preparing to return to my junior year at the University of Pennsylvania, I was stricken with bulbar polio. I was totally paralyzed and unable to breathe without the help of an iron lung. I spent two years in the hospital. I shudder to think how different my life would have been without the determination, guidance and inspiration afforded me by Florence Stattel. She was a tremendous influence in my life and I will be eternally grateful. (Goldberg letter Stattel, October 1997, West Palm Beach, Florida, Stattel private papers)

Florence Stattel (1916–2002), whose biographical sketch is in the 1956 *Who's Who Among American Women*, entered the community of therapists through the Philadelphia School of Occupational Therapy in the 1930s. Unlike her peers and old guard members Crampton, Welles, and West, Stattel entered occupational therapy training without a baccalaureate degree from a more privileged private women's college or university. Like community members Yerxa and Fidler, Stattel's lifelong passion for reading contributed to her professional aspirations and exploring mind. Stattel remembered:

> When I was a little girl my mother's good friend supplied me with books. There was another educated woman who guided my reading. Those were the two women, plus my mother, who said you can be whatever you want. (Stattel/Peters oral history, November 20–21, 1997, lines 289–295)

As an acquaintance of Stattel's five years before her death, I experienced her guiding hand toward my reading choices, continuing this female mentoring process. She was excited and stimulated about occupational therapy's future and the books she read. Our correspondence and conversations reflected her desire to mentor younger women into the community of therapists. Regarding my study, Stattel wrote me:

> Your 1950 through 1980 time frame is good. The news that trained historians [that] are guiding your thinking and expanding the broader health care history in post-World War II is splendid. It is the period that rehabilitation emerged and occupational therapy flourished. Mary [Reilly], Carlotta [Welles] and Willie [West] were classmates and graduates of the Boston School of Occupational Therapy. I served on the AOTA board with Mary Reilly and had her army students. Col. Ruth Robinson was also a

Boston graduate, president of AOTA in the 1950s, and a splendid individual. There is so much that swirls about all these people and the roles they played to advance OT, it is difficult to share on paper. If a note to Mary, Carlotta or Florence is needed, I am happy to oblige. This is an exciting period of 2000 and involved in an evolving profession. At 82, it is a combination of reflections and visionary thinking culled from wisdom distilled from experience that is a thrill as one views the present and future. (Stattel to Peters letter, November 23, 1998, Peters private collection)

In general, she knew about social connections, having been reared in an upper-middle class family. One of seven siblings raised on an 82 acre fruit farm in Kings Park, Long Island, New York, she identified herself as a naturalist, loving animals (Joe, 1998). Having an early health care interest stemming from childhood circumstances, occupational therapy seemed a good fit. Stattel relayed:

Mother was very concerned with infectious disease because two daughters had died, one of diphtheria and the other of polio. I came home with lice in my hair from school, and mother said I was being sent to Catholic school in North Park. I decided I wanted to do a commercial course. I went to the WPA to work for 3 months in 1934. I learned about occupational therapy from high school friend Elizabeth Cusack. Uncle George and Aunt Lotty said 'go down to the Philadelphia School' and they could help with the arrangements.[27] (Stattel/Peters oral history, November 20–21, 1997, lines 101–117; 124–127)

Remembering the Philadelphia School and friend Frieda Behlen, a Philadelphia School alumnus and 1942 New York University occupational therapy chairperson, Stattel said:

I entered the Philadelphia School of Occupational Therapy in 1936 at the age of 19. Graduates of the Philadelphia School of Occupational Therapy in 1939 were taught that occupational therapy is a method of treatment prescribed and guided, with the definite purpose of contributing to and hastening recovery from injury and illness. In 1939 there were 672 OTRs [occupational therapists, registered], today more than 40,000. My starting salary in 1939 was $1,200 a year compared to $4,229 for doctors.

Frieda [Behlen] was my supervisor in 1939. We shared the same desire to help serve humanity through occupational therapy. Her sincerity and directness of purpose opened the way to testing theory with the cooperation of physician and patient. This was the early foundation of the researched practice of today. (Stattel, keynote presentation, unpublished paper, New York University, Department of Occupational Therapy, June 14, 1998)

Stattel's reflections highlight the early 1940s through early 1960s mind-set that occupational therapists worked with physicians cooperatively, if not in an ancillary fashion. Few in the community, except the most independent members like Fidler, Mosey, Ayres, and Yerxa saw themselves as social scientists. This was understandable in the context of the time, and abetted by the nature of occupational therapists. Therapists like Stattel, coming from upper-middle class, white America, were proper young women who spoke up to rather than speak out against, or challenge, male physicians. Demonstrating an appropriate timidity toward men, Stattel talked about how she faced new situations at the Philadelphia School occupational therapy clinic, stating:

> I was in the clinic working with Clare Spackman. One patient, a Black man, said he used to work in the circus and could eat light bulbs. I didn't know whether to tell Clare, I didn't know how to handle it. I had to change from being a shy person to saying this is not permitted in this shop [occupational therapy clinic]. Women didn't talk that way to men whether they were Black or White. I was confronted with things immediately in front of me. (Stattel/Peters oral history, November 20–21, 1997, lines 250–255)

Connected through her Philadelphia School roots and community insiders Willard and Spackman, Stattel served as AOTA's vice president under Willard in 1958. Assuming authority, Stattel developed into a dynamic and forceful professional commanding respect. For example as assistant director of occupational therapy at Kings County Hospital in New York in the late 1940s, she remembered:

> I was arguing with Dr. Deaver at Rusk because he said OTs don't know anything. At Kings County the orthopedic doctors knew we had anatomy and kinesiology, that was different. Bea Wade played a very important part because she knew all the doctors in Chicago. (Stattel/Peters oral history, November 20–21, 1997, lines 4,428–4,439)

Exhausted from career demands, she thought about leaving occupational therapy. Stattel explained:

> I left Connecticut exhausted and went down to Florida.[28] I was approached to go into business, the Ruth Boyle shop on Miracle Mile in Coral Gables, Florida. But after much input from students, I decided I was better staying in occupational therapy.
> I got a call from Frieda who came up with a job doing a research project at Jersey City Medical Center for people with chest disease (Stattel/Peters oral history, November 20–21, 1997, lines 550–555)

Stattel, like others in the community, mixed her professional and social life with other insiders. Traveling to the University of Southern California in 1950 to take a dissection anatomy course, she recounted touring California with other community members while we viewed her 8 mm home movies, saying:

> This is Yosemite and the cottages that Henrietta [Mc Nary] and I stayed in at camp. Freida [Behlen], Henrietta and I had been walking along with Mrs. Behlen [Freida's mother] when we looked up and there was a bear in front of us. The three of us ran. (Stattel/Peters oral history, November 20–21, 1997, lines 37–43)

Earning a Bachelor of Science degree in Occupational Therapy in 1945, and a Master of Arts degree in 1949 in Vocational Rehabilitation at New York University, she worked in clinical and academic settings following new occupational therapy paths. Most notably, she worked as New York City's regional rehabilitation services coordinator from January 1964 until July 1970, where she coordinated state and city rehabilitation services in eight hospitals.

Concerned about staffing shortages, she sent reports to Senator Jacob K. Javits of New York who sat on the Senate Committee on Labor and Public Welfare under Lister Hill's chairmanship in the U.S. Senate. Javits thanked Stattel for her work and looked for future reports (Javits to Stattel letter, United States Senate, November 8, 1968, Stattel private papers). She served on the New York City Regional Interdepartmental Rehabilitation Committee involving herself in medical and health research. In 1969 she was the project director for the New York State Health Department's Bureau of Medical Rehabilitation.

An experienced therapist working in rehabilitation, she began her five-year alliance with physician Henry Kessler at the Kessler Institute for Rehabilitation where she was director of occupational therapy and vocational rehabilitation from 1950 until 1955. Inspired, she wrote about the hospital, and patients with phantom limb syndrome, amputations, and about equipment design, which was the subject of her Eleanor Clarke Slagle lecture (Stattel, 1952, 1954, 1956). Stattel was the first recipient of the 1955 Eleanor Clarke Slagle lectureship, indicating her respect from peers and her contributions. Acknowledging occupational therapy philosophical and scientific knowledge in her Slagle lecture she said:

> Occupational therapy had its conception in the faith and conviction of our early founders. It developed as a profession because of strong beliefs. We have been given a wonderful professional heritage of courage and wisdom and as we continue to extend our hand to benefit mankind; may we continue to believe and search for further knowledge. (Stattel, F. M., 1956, p. 194)

Stattel's academic appointments included associate professor at the University of Florida, Gainesville (1971–1972); and Texas Woman's University (1972–1975). Stattel was interested in occupational therapy's past and how it fit into a changing society. On occupational therapy's 60th anniversary, Stattel asked whether "we are ready to commit research, documentation and publication of a comprehensive history of occupational therapy in the United States to top priority" (1977, p. 650) She further questioned, "In the absence of a comprehensive history, can we have a historical perspective and understanding of the past to consider as a resource for continuity planning?" (p. 650). Stattel (1966) linked future planning to new occupational therapy knowledge and a larger rehabilitation work force. Seeing a bright 1960s outlook, she suggested:

> We can move ahead on the mainstream of the present national effort, propelled by our society's concern for human services. Despite the gravity and complexity of their problems, occupational therapists, along with other trained medical health rehabilitation personnel will find new uses and purposes for themselves. They will sit together and work out solutions to common problems and will assess the past and accept the inevitable changes. (Stattel, 1966, p. 146)

In the same light she stated:

> To remain in the mainstream of social action, occupational therapists must be tuned into the changes that lie ahead. The practicing occupational therapist is perhaps more aware of the need for facts that provide justification for practice. Change, which reached record speed in the 50 s, has moved to the point where assessments must be made yearly. This means that the present is rapidly accruing a past that in volume and scope is staggering to comprehend. (Stattel, private papers, June 1976, East Hampton, New York).

In 1998, Stattel received AOTA's Award of Merit because she was viewed as an occupational therapy "pioneer" (AOTA, 1998b, p. 12). Receiving her award in Baltimore, Maryland on April 4, 1998, she summed up her career, stating:

> Occupational therapy has a universal message that has received acceptance. Emphasis is on the mind and body, how they develop when in harmony, to produce purposeful activity. I am honored to be the first Eleanor Clarke Slagle lecturer and an Award of Merit recipient, a lifelong member of AOTA, a Charter member of the World Federation of Occupational Therapists and a supporting member of the American Occupational Therapy Foundation.[29] The letters OTR [occupational therapist registered] are an indelible part of my professional and self-identity, and the Good Lord has been my mentor. (Stattel private papers, 1998)

Similarly, and more controversially, she stated:

> I think we have been a mixture of always questioning who we are. Personally I don't think that is bad. I think to live is to change, we must

look at our systems. We must retain what we felt. We were humanitarians; we were concerned with the whole person. Our strength is coming and working with other people. We should not lose the humanitarian spirit. We should not become academics; this is my big concern. (Stattel/Peters oral history, November 20–21, 1997, lines 640–644, 653–654)

Stattel's reflections about occupational therapy's purpose and her commitment to its existence exemplify the beliefs and actions of an old-guard sustainer. Characterizing herself, Stattel said: "I was an idealist. I never knew where occupational therapy would take me," (Stattel/Peters oral history, November 20–21, 1997, line 237). She continued to raise questions about occupational therapy's future, including a student scholarship loan program in her name at AOTF. AOTF Executive Director Kirkland stated, "Florence is a woman with a grand vision for occupational therapy. Her ideas are as fresh and inspiring today as they were decades ago when she first began writing about the future of the profession," (Joe, 1998, p. 14).

Carlotta Welles, a contemporary of Marion Crampton and Florence Stattel, is the last old-guard community sustainer discussed. Crampton, a Bostonian, and Stattel a New Yorker, represent East Coast therapists, whereas Welles is a Los Angeles therapist, providing some insight into California's developing think tank.

Carlotta Welles

Carlotta Welles, an occupational therapist for more than 60 years, with a special interest in occupational therapy ethics and liability (Welles, 1969, 1976, 1979, 1984, 1985), administration (Welles, 1962) and rehabilitation (Welles, 1952, 1958), embodies the concepts of an old guard sustainer and community insider. A down-to-earth woman, she characterized herself in the following passage, stating:

> The basic part of me is that I know how to manage money because I had a very strict allowance that I have always managed well. The next thing is that I am very mechanical, and that's how I got into OT. (Welles/Peters oral history, April 28–29, 2003, lines 3,440–3,444)

Welles statement parallels community member Fidler, who like Welles was most attracted to occupational therapy's activity base rather than the idea of helping people with disabilities as a primary motivator. Like Fidler, she questioned occupational therapy's knowledge-based development, and the profession's status, asking: "Is occupational therapy still a simple, elementary discipline?" (Welles, 1958, p. 290). Welles, a proponent of specialized knowledge, believed that there was a widespread feeling that "our present practice is no longer adequate" (Welles, 1958, p. 290).

Concerned about increasing her own occupational therapy knowledge, she interrupted her established career and enrolled in the University of Southern California graduate program full-time. The University of Southern California offered the first Master's Degree in Occupational Therapy in the early 1950s. Earning her Master of Arts degree in 1953 alongside Cromwell, and shortly after first graduate West, she stated her reason for pursuing her graduate degree, saying:

> I wanted to teach, and I thought it would further my career all the way around. I thought people who want to get somewhere write. I needed to express my finding(s) to other people. I didn't write for the credit that I would get. I thought a professional person should be known in the literature. I could have done better work with a doctorate. (Welles/Peters oral history, April 28–29, 2003, lines 3,545–3,557; 3,574–3,578; 6,958–6,960)

Welles was and is a major occupational therapy contributor, providing her talents and financial resources anonymously as acknowledged in her Honorary Life Membership to AOTF's Board of Directors since 1994. The mechanically- killed Welles remembers her first thoughts about occupational therapy by stating:

> I was always building things. I got into OT because I thought I could keep working with tools and helping other people with tools. I didn't realize the amount of medical work it turned out to be. (Welles/Peters oral history, August 28–29, 2003, lines 3,447–3,451)

Welles understood medical limitations, although she denied that this knowledge had anything to do with her choosing occupational therapy. Her father retired early because of health issues, and she watched her younger sister adjust to childhood rheumatic fever. Welles stated:

> My father wasn't well, but he kept going. I have a younger sister Lou. When she was little she had rheumatic fever for years and years. She had a nurse, and everything was first for my sister. I hated that. Tools were my refuge. I had a little room that I called my workshop. (Welles/Peters oral history, April 28–29, 2003, lines 3,680–3,683; 3,702–3,716)

Welles, raised in Alta Dena, California, came to occupational therapy immediately after her 1939 Scripps College graduation in California. Welles was the type of young woman occupational therapy educational program directors sought: a well-educated, cultured, upper-class, white women like they were. Her society-oriented mother maintained her Brookline, Massachusetts connections while exposing her two daughters to upper-class values and expectations. Returning during summers to New England, the Welles family sailed and exposed their daughters to their deep

Massachusetts and Connecticut roots. Explaining her *Who's Who Among American Women* registry, Welles was discreet about her background:

> Education was very important, but also contributing to society. I'm reluctant to say, but my family was prominent in Pasadena. I didn't want to ride on their coattails. They were a generous family. They taught us to take care of our money, and that some of it must be given away.
>
> I'm a Colonial Dame and sit on their board.[30] It sounds snobby, but you have to have a colonial ancestor and be socially acceptable, and mother saw to that. I've never told anyone, but I had a coming out party, a cotillion. Mother was a Boston lady who went to Smith. She didn't have a career outside the home because you didn't then. She volunteered at a crippled children's place in Brookline, and was very literary, into classics and music. We spoke several languages, all of us. I was expected to learn French. My sister and I worked in Normandy [France] in a camp for underprivileged children. We ran an activity program with nothing, and right after the war we left.
>
> I was very attached to my father, who was an engineer. He went to Amherst and then MIT [Massachusetts Institute of Technology]. Our home was like an engineering place. I admired him greatly, so I had tools, and used tools, and we used tools together. (Welles/Peters oral history, April 28–29, 2003, lines 153–154; 4,132–4,137; 168–170; 3,323–3,284; 4,122–4,218; 526–543; 4,230–4,256; 1,298–1,304; 93–158)

Welles' mechanical aptitude in using carpentry tools led her to occupational therapy rather than engineering. Similar to younger community member Gilfoyle's narrative, Welles believed that women were excluded from engineering programs. Graduating with a liberal arts degree from an exclusive private women's college may have been enough for other women in her generation, but Welles sought more. She explained how she enrolled in the BSOT, stating:

> I've always liked tools, and from the time I was little I had tools. A distant cousin knew about occupational therapy, it sounded just right, hardly knowing what it was. I was charmed because of the tools; the people relationships didn't enter my mind. I was going to have a profession with tools. I went and applied at the Boston School with mother. In the fall of '39 I enrolled and finished in '41. It didn't give degrees because it had no university connection at the time; it gave diplomas." (Welles/Peters oral history, April 28–29, 2003, lines 68–147; 156–160)

Welles was one of 11 graduates of the BSOT in 1941 (AOTF Connection, 1998, p. 1). She sat next to classmate Wilma West, beginning their lifelong friendship and mutual belief in occupational therapy's contribution to society. Recalling West, Welles stated:

> We went to the same school at the same time. Being 'W' 'E' we sat side-by-side because we were seated alphabetically. We knew each other

very well. I enjoyed her very much. She came and visited my family, and came on the boat without great success. Willie came from a different background than I did. My parents didn't accept her. Her family ran a farm,[31] and my family, through no special virtue, were the leading citizens in the town. Willie knew only farming. OT was a new world to her. She was a reliable and good person. (Welles/Peters oral history, April 28–29, 2003, lines 3,224–3,250)

As a West peer, Welles was on equal community footing and influential. Recognized for her leadership contributions, she received AOTA's Award of Merit in 1975 during Jerry Johnson's AOTA presidency. In 1992, she received AOTA and AOTF's President's Commendation in honor of Wilma West. I was present when she accepted the honor at AOTA's 1992 conference as she stood proudly next to her life companion and occupational therapy leader, Florence Cromwell. Welles thanked the profession and Cromwell for a fulfilling professional and personal life. Welles spoke about first meeting Cromwell, stating:

> I was lucky to get her for training at the General Hospital in Los Angeles as a student in 1949. I kept her, and that was 54 years ago. We built a house in Pasadena, we had dogs, we traveled, we went on the boat, and we camped. (Welles/Peters oral history, April 28–29, 2003, lines 435–437; 553–577)

Cromwell acknowledged how Welles, 15 years her senior, mentored and introduced her to many occupational therapists whom she referred to as Carlotta's friends. When one is as well-placed as Welles, friendships meant community ties. Welles discussed some peers and Award of Merit recipients: Kahmann, Robinson, Gleave, Kilburn, Crampton, and Spackman. They served on AOTA and AOTF boards of management together, as well as on the following committees: graduate study, clinical research, standards for the profession, personnel, and fiscal advisory. Remembering the community like a montage, Welles stated:

> I've had people that I admired, but I don't think I had anybody that specially looked out for me. I knew Connie [Kahmann] quite well; I was on committees with her. I didn't imitate everything, for example she drank, but I wanted to learn from her. Ruth Robinson was one of the presidents, and she and I were very good friends. Ruth was generous in relating to people, giving them credit. Maggie Gleave was a marvelous committee person with a great strength in clinical education. She was a neat person, and the head of OT at Cleveland Children's Hospital. Clare [Spackman] was there [clinical training committee] too. Crampy [Crampton] was a friend. I remember Ginny Kilburn. She supervised the workshop and students at the Philadelphia School, but there's not much to say about her.[32] (Welles/Peters oral history, April 28–29, 2003, lines 4,439–4,448; 3,793–3,803; 3,200–3,213; 3,826–3,885; 3,868–3,673)

Welles worked primarily in California, except for the period 1955 to 1956, when she worked on curriculum design and taught at the Philadelphia School of Occupational Therapy with Willard and Spackman; and her first position in 1942 was at Hartford Hospital in Hartford, Connecticut. From 1944 to 1946, Welles, a capable administrator, worked for the United States Army in a civilian capacity. Her peers, Kahmann, West, and Reilly, who made occupational therapy military decisions, communicated easily with Welles. She recounted her military years in the following autobiographical paragraphs:

> In 1942, when the Army began requesting occupational therapists for military hospital duty, I volunteered in a civilian role. Later we were made the Womens Medical Specialist Corps, with physical therapists and dieticians. There were 800 occupational therapists in 40 Army hospitals. The Corps was gradually integrated into the military, some physical therapists and dieticians were sent overseas, but OTs were not.
>
> I was chief occupational therapist at Birmingham Army Hospital, in Van Nuys, California. I employed 14 occupational therapists and 40 volunteers to serve the 1,200-bed hospital population. Our volunteers, most from the nearby movie community, added much. Mary Astor and Walter Wanger came regularly. Charles Laughton read the Bible and Shakespeare to patients. I was transferred to Fort Douglas [Headquarters, Ninth Service Command] in Salt Lake City and made supervisor of the entire West Coast, which had 10 hospitals and 160 therapists. The chief of occupational therapy [Kahmann] and I were good friends. I phoned her directly if we had problems. (Welles Army Medical Specialist Corp Presentation, May 1999, Welles private papers)

From 1947 to 1953, Welles directed the occupational therapy department at Los Angeles County General Hospital where Cromwell was assistant chief of occupational therapy. Training many students, including Yerxa, Welles and Cromwell worked well together. Invested in occupational therapy education, Welles spent 1968–1978 as the founding chairperson of the Los Angeles City College Occupational Therapy Assistant Educational Program prior to retirement.

Summarizing her career, Welles portrayed herself as a hard worker and involved therapist. She stated:

> I had a number of papers [journal articles]. I like to be known in what I do. I was a board member, and I was a delegate [AOTA Delegate Assembly]. I don't just work off in a corner like a pit mouse. I go to things and meet people. (Welles/Peters oral history, April 28–29, 2003, lines 3,553–3,557)

Welles' words express how community insiders, and sustainers, functioned. They provided the infrastructure and resources to continue supporting occupational therapy's existence.

Therapists Crampton, Stattel, and Welles typified occupational therapy's old-guard sustainers. Completing their occupational therapy education within a three-year time frame, Crampton and Welles earned their BSOT certificates in 1938 and 1941 respectively, and Stattel was a 1939 Philadelphia School of Occupational Therapy certificate graduate. They observed 65 years of occupational therapy's progress from the insider's perspective. Knowing each other, working side-by-side on AOTA and AOTA committees, they contributed a gracious and privileged upper-class professional tone that supported all community members' belief in occupational therapy's worth.

Robert K. Bing and Lela A. Llorens represent occupational therapy's new guard sustainers who supported the profession and broke new minority barriers.

Robert K. Bing

Examining Robert K. Bing's (1929–2003) private papers shortly after his death, I noted that he was a man who enjoyed, studied, preserved, and wrote about occupational therapy's past (Bing, 1981, 1983a, 1983b, 1984a, 1984b, 1993, 1997). Referred to as Bob by his peers, he lectured and wrote about occupational therapy's history. Most notably in his 1981 Slagle lecture, Bing introduced his audience to William Tuke, Benjamin Rush, Adolf Meyer, George Barton, Susan Tracy, William Rush Dunton, Jr., and Eleanor Clarke Slagle, whose ideas shaped occupational therapy. He stated:

> This is a statement of how an idea, born in a philosophical movement, became activated through the good works of men and women who inalterably believed in the ideal that those who are sick and handicapped can regain, retain, and attain some semblance of function within the fundamental limitations of the human organism and the expectations of society in which all must exist: that this may occur through the most obvious means of all—one's reorganization through occupation, through activity, through leisure, and through rest. This journey about occupational therapy, its evolution and development presents vexation: one must accept a fair number of ambiguities, something some today consider a fundamental problem in occupational therapy. (Bing, 1981, AJOT, p. 500).

Bing's thought that founders believed in an ideal originating in philosophy parallels this community of therapists' common belief in occupational therapy's value and its societal contribution, and hints at the debate about a philosophic, rather than a scientific, foundation.

Being graduated in 1952 with a Bachelor of Science Degree in Occupational Therapy from the University of Illinois, Bing entered the community of therapists through the auspices of his academic program director and old-guard insider, Beatrice Wade. He retired in 1989 as Professor Emeritus, University of Texas Medical Branch, Galveston, from his position as the Dean of the School of Allied Health Sciences, which he had held since 1968. He characterized his career shift, stating:

> I became more involved in educational administration and less in practice. I remained very active in OT, and gained different kinds of perspectives about what was developing in the profession when compared with other comparable groups such as PT [physical therapy], medical technology, and the physician's assistant. (Bing/Peters oral history, January 31, 2003, lines 14–18)

Gaining a new perspective as a dean, and establishing the first school of allied health in the Southwest, Bing presented his thoughts in "Requisites for Relevance," suggesting occupational therapists think about education with an eye on the changing health care delivery system. He stated:

> I have moved away from a single orientation, that of occupational therapy, toward a more eclectic approach in relation to the education of the young health professional. If occupational therapy, along with other health-related professions is to survive and thrive in the present and future atmosphere of the "push-pull-click-click" of health care services, then it must remain relevant (Bing, 1969a).

Perhaps controversial, Bing (1969b) predicted the emergence of a more generic health care professional. He received the profession's highest honors, including AOTA's Eleanor Clarke Slagle Lectureship in 1981, and AOTA's Award of Merit in 1987. Bing was the first and only male occupational therapist elected AOTA president and served from 1983–1986. Breaking new barriers as a part of his new-guard sustainer status, at times he faced community resistance from other occupational therapy leaders. Bing, as a male therapist in a predominantly female profession, candidly stated "I am going to bare my soul and reveal 'family secrets,' some of it a bit scandalous, considering the times. I am willing to own my thoughts." (Bing/Peters oral history, February 6, 2003, lines 20–28).

It is hard to determine whether his male status in a predominantly female profession worked against him, or whether some just did not appreciate his singular contributions. Remembering gender differences, Bing recounted attending his first AOTA conference in Washington, DC, portraying the 1950s crafts-oriented therapist. He recalled:

> My first conference was in Washington, DC, at the old Sheraton in the Park, fall 1954. I was a new faculty member at Richmond Professional Institute [now Virginia Commonwealth University]. I wandered around a couple of hours trying to soak in the culture. I was shocked. Most of the ladies were middle age and above. They were enwrapped in homemade knitted and crocheted shawls, and many of them had "cutesie"

crocheted hats, some with pipe cleaners coming out the tops looking something like flowers. In meetings, several ladies had brought their hobbies with them, knitting, crocheting, needlepointing as the speakers droned. I wondered what had I gotten myself into. There were just a handful of men, relatively few young people my age, in the mid-late 20 s. Most of these had to stay home and look after patients while supervisors and chiefs came to conference. (Bing/Peters oral history, February 11, 2003, lines 173–189)

The image that Bing colorfully portrayed stereotyped supervisory occupational therapists as crafts ladies rather than laboratory coat scientists and professionals. Examining photographs from the 1950s, guest presenters and occupational therapy leaders wore conservative suits with well-manicured hair; however, Bing's picture of a handicrafts-toting therapist is a tradition that continues in the culture. What Bing raises is a question about what impression this makes to outsiders; did the 1950s membership present a professional image of authority?

Feeling like an outsider, Bing recalled his presidential election 30 years after that 1950s AOTA conference, stating:

I think of how the news of my becoming president-elect absolutely underwhelmed people. The official announcement came near the end of the annual business meeting in Philadelphia. Not one soul came up to me to congratulate me or extend best wishes, or tell me that I was an absolute sucker. I simply was left standing there. I walked out of the hotel and sat down in a lovely little park that had lots of flowers. I sat an hour internalizing my feelings. I had some doubts about whether I really wanted to do this, but felt I needed to soldier on. The total lack of response had me wonder[ing] if that was the kind of ennui I would face from the membership. It was, throughout my term. I heard from people when they wanted something to advance their own agenda. (Bing/Peters oral history, March 3, 2003, lines 1,135–1,149)

Community members Cromwell, Fidler, Gilfoyle, and Welles shared their impression about Bing's presidency. Their comments showed that Bing's reservations held some painful truth.

Fidler: "Bob is a character onto himself. He has always been controversial in many ways and that was very well known." (Fidler/Peters oral history, March 6–7, 2003, lines 7,375–7,390)

Gilfoyle: "I looked at Bob Bing as president, and didn't see him carry out leadership." (Gilfoyle/Peters oral history, February 10–11, 2003, lines 2,106–2,108)

Cromwell: "We didn't have any men presidents until Bob Bing who always wanted to be president. He was the weakest link in the chain. He was professorial and that was his avenue in life.

He was a sweet guy, but he never set the world on fire. Those are my own feelings." (Cromwell/Peters oral history, April 28–29, 2003, lines 5,861–5,870)

Welles: "I liked him and was on a committee with him. He was quiet and gentle, but it didn't get him ahead. He'd never set the world on fire." (Welles/Peters oral history, April 28–29, 2003, lines 5,881–5,889)

These occupational therapy leaders portrayed one side but not a complete story, and in certain situations he didn't feel any animosity. For example, he remembered transitioning AOTA's presidency to Gilfoyle, stating "Ellie (Gilfoyle) succeeded me as president of AOTA. We served together and got along quite well." (Bing/Peters oral history, February 17, 2003, lines 289–292)

Bing's career long protégé relationship with strong insider Beatrice Wade guided his community course, as illustrated in the following:

Bea was an advocate of volunteerism, which was the life blood of any organization. She also believed that volunteers needed mentors and time to develop. Once she had completed her task, she would hand you on to someone who could help you to the next level. In my case it was Mary Alice Coombs, a graduate of the old school at Shepphard–Pratt Hospital, Towson, Maryland.[33] Mary Alice introduced me to Dr. William Rush Dunton. (Bing/Peters oral history, January 30, 2003, lines 5–11)

Bing, drafted as a private during the Korean conflict near the end of his occupational therapy education, remembered Wade's insider actions at another time in his life:

The 50s were my formative years. I graduated from the University of Illinois in 1952, having first enrolled in 1949. The draft board sent me off to the army in mid July 1951. Bea Wade, my school director, was appalled that nothing was being done to salvage me.

She got in touch with the chief of OT in the Army and told her the situation. She, in turn, very quietly rearranged assignment rosters, so I was allowed to complete the 6 months of clinical training. (Bing/Peters oral history, February 11, 2003, lines 224–240)

A second Bing supporter, occupational therapy promoter and physician William Rush Dunton, Jr., became the subject for his University of Maryland doctoral dissertation. Bing explained:

Of all my OT experiences, my connection to Dr. Dunton has had the most profound impact. I came to adore that man in his early 90s. What richness happens when you have a mentoring system.[34] (Bing/Peters oral history, January 30, 2003, lines 10–11, February 6, 2003, lines 120–121)

While living in Maryland, Bing formed a collegial friendship with community insider Ruth Brunyate Wiemer, who was close to Dunton. Maintaining his community relationships, Bing, while a Dean at the University of Texas, Galveston, established a yearly visiting occupational therapy scholar and leaders lectureship. Weimer remembered her guest lecture, viewing a photograph, stating "That is a picture of me at the University of Texas in 1972; I was one of the class sponsors." (Wiemer/Peters oral history, March 18–19, 2003, lines 4,016–4,023)

Today at the University of Texas, a portrait of Bing hangs in the Allied Health Building. There is also the Robert K. Bing Scholars Program in the Department of Occupational Therapy, which provides financial assistance to an occupational therapy student with more than a $66,000 endowment (Robert K. Bing Scholars Program; http://www.sahs.utmb.edu/giving.asp, 2/26/2002).

Having community connections like Wade, Dunton, and Wiemer, it is perplexing that Bing seriously thought about leaving occupational therapy. Teaching at the University of Florida, Gainesville, from 1961 until 1963, as assistant professor of occupational therapy, he experienced a difficult working relationship with department chairperson Alice Jantzen. Jantzen, a member of the Jantzen swimsuit family and a Wellesley and BSOT graduate, was a well-connected community member. Bing described a tumultuous relationship, which ending disappointingly, stating:

> I received a letter from Alice [Jantzen] saying that I would not be reappointed the following year. I was being fired. I made an appointment with the dean who felt he could ease Alice out and then appoint me chair. The next day I submitted my resignation. During the summer I was scheduled to be a faculty member at a psychiatric OT workshop in Chicago with Mary Alice Coombs. I told Mary Alice that I would be teaching human development in the fall of 1963 in the College of Education at the University of Maryland. I was getting out of OT altogether. I felt whipped. (Bing/Peters oral history, February 17, 2003, lines 440–463)

He returned to his clinical work in psychiatry as the director of activity therapy, Illinois State Psychiatric Institute, Chicago, with a dual appointment as assistant professor of occupational therapy at University of Illinois, College of Medicine, Chicago in 1963. Remotivated, Bing remembered; "I spent two days being interviewed and I particularly liked the idea of building a clinical education program," (Bing/Peters oral history, February 17, 2003, lines 468–470. Preparing a staff handbook titled "Methods of Research for the Occupational Therapist," he introduced various research techniques he categorized as historical, observational, case study, questionnaire, interview, survey, and experimental research. His handwritten notes showed his interest in linking research to practice (Bing, 1954, 1958, 1961, 1962, 1987, private papers).

Bing's professional career continued to have high and low points. Sharing his patriot pride by wearing a Texas state pin on his lapel, Bing wrote about his unique experience attending President Reagan's signing ceremony for the Proclamation of the Decade of Disabled Persons at the White House, November 28, 1983. Bing wrote:

> November 28th was a cool and rainy day in Washington as I drove through the streets that are so familiar to every American. As I reflect on my experiences of that morning, I was honored to be in the presence of the President [Reagan] and Vice President [Bush], but as an occupational therapist I was more impressed that a document promising a national 10-year commitment to improving life for the disabled of our country was afforded attention approaching that of our efforts toward achieving world peace. (AOTA, 1984, pp. 1, 10).

Bing, a Nebraska-born American who grew up in Cape Girardeau, Missouri, never envisioned a White House invitation. A devoutly religious practicing Unitarian, and of German American heritage, Bing never married. Attached to both parents, Bing emulated his father's academic teaching career path. His father was an industrial arts professor at East Carolina University, and in the summers of 1950 and 1958 Bing took additional classes there. Saving his father's technical drawings and course syllabi, his industrial arts skills transferred easily to occupational therapy. Bing discussed his parents' influence, stating:

> I came from a family of educators and I knew that I should get at least a master's. But in what? On weekends I sat for hours in the Denver Public Library.[35] The University of Maryland had an Institute for Child Study designed for teachers. I wrote the Institute and told them I wanted to study children since I had had very little in my undergraduate days. Miss Wade thought it would be inappropriate for a young man to work with kids. I was surprised to receive an invitation to work on the doctorate. The dissertation became a family enterprise. We went through Dad's first, then mine. My mother played the important role as grammarian, typist and all-around clock watcher, insisting that we get the job done. (Bing/Peters oral history, February 11, 2003, lines 249–266, February 22, 2003, lines 606–610)

In the previous passage, Bing alluded to Miss Wade's belief that male occupational therapists should not work with children. This stereotype shaped a potential practice and research area for Bing. Bing's 1954 Master of Arts thesis; "A study of pediatric adjustment methods and techniques in a select group of hospitals," was his attempt to break barriers. The community of therapists perpetuated gender bias as reflected in the following passages. For example, Fidler stated:

> OTs feel inadequate, and men feel doubly inadequate. A very different kind of man, typically a blue-collar man or those from uneducated families came into occupational therapy seeking upward mobility. Women do not look so much for upward mobility. They look for opportunities to take care of people. Neither is conducive to scientific inquiry. Looking at research is not part of the picture. Male therapists want the education in a hurry so they can make money. (Fidler/Peters oral history, March 6–7, 2003, lines 4,689–4,701, 1,616–1,638)

True to Fidler's profile, Bing did pursue an administrative career; however, his family was educated, contradicting the blue-collar statement. Secondly, Bing contributed to occupational therapy's body of knowledge.

Like Fidler, community member Cromwell thought male therapists had some unfair advantages while desiring and achieving an administrative fast track. Cromwell stated:

> The men that we have attracted, by and large are not strong people. They're not strong personalities; they're not strong administrators. Some of them are real nice guys. They probably had a fast line to admission, because they knew they wanted to get them into OT school. Women vote for men if they run for anything. (Cromwell/Peters oral history, April 28–29, 2003, lines 6,746–6752; 6,781–6,792).

Contrasted with Fidler's, Yerxa's, and Cromwell's reflections, Bing struggled at times, feeling like an occupational therapy minority, and one without advantages or privilege. These feelings motivated his continued education. He stated:

> 'White men come with privilege' does not square with a white male in a female population. Maybe that is what was taking place with me, as I continued to advance up the academic ladder, including my doctorate. I became more 'privileged' and less vulnerable to scratching and clawing. It was my armor. (Bing/Peters oral history, April 24, 2003, lines 1,353–1,357)

He remembered sharing feelings of separateness with African American female occupational therapy leader and scholar, Lela A. Llorens, the next community member discussed, and Marian Ross, who also contributed to the profession. Bing stated:

> During my presidential years, I talked a lot with Lee Llorens and Marian Ross about being minorities in OT. They seemed to feel that they were

specially picked to go to OT school because they showed great promise, and that White directors tended to believe that it was the 'right thing to do.' It was a fairness issue. (Bing/Peters oral history, April 24, 2003, lines 1,358–1,364)

Identifying as a minority, Bing paralleled his experience as a male occupational therapist to racial barriers that he felt Black therapists faced. He remembered an unanticipated experience accepting an invitation to AOTA's yearly Black Caucus meeting at conference while he was president elect in 1982, saying:

Sometime in the 70 s the Black Caucus was created. I was invited to meet with them and say welcome. I sat down thinking I would be staying for the meeting. 'Oh no, you are only here to say hello.' Who knows what goes on in there? The executive board never received a report from the caucus. I always thought that was peculiar. (Bing/Peters oral history, April 24, 2003, lines 1,368–1,373)

Bing did not clarify whether he was informed that the meeting was closed to non-group members, or whether his official capacity as president elect warranted his perceived exclusion. Taking episodes like this personally, Bing stated he felt his efforts weren't appreciated. However misunderstood in the community, including short teaching tenures at Richmond Professional Institute, Richmond, Virginia (1954–1956), the University of Florida, Gainesville (1961–1963), and Elizabethtown College in Elizabethtown, Pennsylvania (1986–1987), Bing shared the belief held by others of occupational therapy's worthwhile-breaking-gender-barriers through his scholarly contributions.

The last community member to be highlighted, Lela A. Llorens, is an occupational therapy scholar and leader who also symbolized community change, introducing the new-guard dimension.

Lela A. Llorens

Lela A. Llorens is an early contributor to occupational therapy's theoretical knowledge who supported occupational therapy practice. She said, "Standing the test of time, people credit me the most with initiating some thought in relationship to theory development" (Llorens/Peters oral history, April 25–26, 2003, lines 3,799–3,802). In her 1969 Eleanor Clarke Slagle Lectureship titled "Facilitating growth and development: The promise of occupational therapy," Llorens presented a developmental theoretical taxonomy. Her thesis was that "occupational therapy is a facilitation process which assists the individual in achieving mastery of life tasks and the ability to cope…, through the mechanisms of selected input stimuli and availability of practice in a suitable environment" (Llorens, 1970, p. 93). Valuing her Slagle lecture-ship, she stated:

> That was a milestone as a professional to be recognized by your peers as having something to say. The lectureship was important to me because intellectual accomplishment is important. It's part of the value system that I grew up with, that education and learning was, and still is, important. It's the highest award for intellectual accomplishment that the field had to offer, and that was more important to me than the Award of Merit that I really appreciated getting. (Llorens/Peters oral history, April 25–26, 2003, lines 2,565–2,583)

A recognized occupational therapy scholar and leader, she contributed countless volunteer hours to the profession. Llorens, developing occupational therapy research efforts in the late 1970s, including reviewing grants, and determining a direction with other committee members like Gilfoyle, Gillette, and Yerxa in the late 1970s, also chaired AOTF's Research Advisory Committee from 1978 until 1989 (AOTA, 1978). West, in her role as foundation president, presenting AOTF's Certificate of Appreciation to Llorens, said:

> Assuming the difficult task of initiating a bold new program in the foundation to implement a mandate from the association for all research in the profession, Lela Llorens, PhD, FAOTA, and OTR extraordinaire, has led the research advisory committee in lengthened strides toward the goal of more and better research in occupational therapy. (American Occupational Therapy Foundation, 1982, The 1981 Certificates of Appreciation, AJOT, p. 195).[36]

Among other awards, Llorens received her AOTA Award of Merit in 1987, AOTF's A. Jean Ayres Award in 1988 for her contributions to the development and application of theory, and she was the fourth recipient of AOTA's and AOTF's President's Commendation in honor of Wilma L. West in 1997. Martha Kirkland, executive director of AOTF, presenting the President's Commendation Award stated:

> We thank her on behalf of her colleagues nationwide who continue to benefit from her vision, leadership, and integrity. Her record of service to her professional community is one of unselfish dedication. In honoring her, we as a professional community, perpetuate the values and principles of one of the profession's greatest leaders, Wilma L. West. (Berg, 1997, p. 16).

Kirkland's words reflect Llorens' community involvement and insider status. Personally knowing West and Ayres and receiving awards in their honor, exemplified her peer group and accomplishments. Prior to her death, West shared her thoughts about their alliance, stating:

> I first became aware of Lela Llorens when her name began appearing on research articles emanating from the Lafayette Clinic in Detroit. That was the early 1960s when few OTs were involved in interdisciplinary teams of research. My literature acquaintance with Lee developed rapidly into a personal friendship and greater collegial admiration in the mid-to late-60 s through firsthand knowledge of her work . . . (West, 1991, p. 10).

West, as she did with other talented therapists, introduced and positioned Llorens in the community of therapists. Perhaps not predicted or intended, Llorens broke new racial ground in the profession's leadership that challenged occupational therapy's White, Anglo Saxon, Protestant roots. Llorens stated:

> I really think that the African American occupational therapists were very proud to have someone in the positions that I have been in, and have been very supportive. By the same token I think that my Caucasian collea-gues have been supportive and proud. I've felt that I could call upon any-one that I needed to do whatever needed to be done. Lawrene Kovalenko once said that I was a citizen of the world. That is how I view myself. (Llorens/Peters oral history, April 25–26, 2003, lines 4,957–5,005)

Sensing a responsibility about her Slagle lecture, Llorens remembered:

> I feared I'd have nothing else to say. That didn't prove to be true, but that was something I worried about. Am I ever going to have anything else to publish? It (the Slagle) meant something to me. (Llorens/Peters oral history, April 25–26, 2003, lines 2,585–2,600)

Progressing past her concerns she remained motivated to answer her own questions about occupational therapy. Similar to other community of therapist members discussed, Llorens strongly believed in occupational therapy and in developing a knowledge base. (Llorens, 1970, 1973, 1974a, 1974b, 1977, 1981a, 1981b, 1984, 1990; Llorens & Synder, 1987). She reflected:

> Some people might have felt some awe about the kinds of things that I was doing because it did take a certain chutzpah. But I didn't think about it that way. To me it was a natural progression. Everything I've done is the next step in a quest for finding out what occupational therapy was about and could do. I wasn't going to give up until I was satisfied that I knew. (Llorens/Peters oral history, April 25–26, 2003, lines 1,010–1,018)

Prior to meeting community leader West, Llorens learned about an old-guard community culture through her academic program director Marion

R. Spear.[37] Remembering her entrance interview with "Miss Spear" at Western Michigan University, Llorens recounted a stressful interview process. Regarding the student who interviewed before her, Llorens stated:

> She [Spear] interviewed all the students before she would admit them into the program. The student feared that she wouldn't be let into the program because she wore a brace and had a crutch. I still remember she left her crutch out in the hall and walked into Miss Spear's office. Because I had been in a program before, I had an easier time being admitted.[38,39] (Llorens/Peters oral history April 25–26, 2003, lines 339–360)

Llorens described Spear's interviewing process using similar words to those of community members Crampton, Fidler, Stattel, Wiemer, Welles, and Yerxa. Cast back to the founding years when white, upper-middle class women entered occupational therapy, the 1950s occupational therapy program directors searched for "proper young women." Llorens talked about 1950s racial considerations that complicated applicant acceptance, saying:

> There aren't a lot of African Americans in occupational therapy, even today. There was sensitivity to the fact that if we let these people in, they won't get jobs. There were places where the people who were recruiting for occupational therapy were trying to protect the students being rejected by patients who wouldn't want an African American working with or on them. (Llorens/Peters oral history, April 25–26, 2003, lines 315–335)

Characterizing herself as one of "Miss Spear's girls," Llorens received the Marion R. Spear Scholastic Award in 1953. She remembered the award's namesake: "You knew what Miss Spear expected from her girls. It wasn't a personal mentorship; it was an expected behavior or a set of social norms." (Llorens/Peters oral history, April 25–26, 2003, lines 787–790)

Llorens was graduated in 1953, at age 20, from Western Michigan University with a Bachelor of Science Degree in Occupational Therapy. Starting her occupational therapy career in 1953 at Wayne County General Hospital, she remembered interviewing for the Lafayette Clinic, where she worked from 1961 until 1968. While conducting research with a multidisciplinary team, including psychiatrists, psychologists, social workers, recreation therapists, art therapists and special educators, Llorens wrote about occupational therapy's scientific contributions in child psychiatry, including single case studies, and testing and treatment intervention. (Llorens, 1960, 1967a, 1967b, 1968a, 1968b, 1972, 1974a, 1974b; Llorens & Bernstein, 1963; Llorens, Lev, & Rubin, 1964; Llorens & Rubin, 1962; Llorens, Rubin, et al., 1964). She remembered:

> The Lafayette Clinic was a research facility. It was elite in the state of Michigan, as it was the only one of its kind. It received funding from the state and from volunteer organizations such as the Junior League.

People were careful who could belong to this club. I wasn't sure I'd get the position because there is snobbery in occupational therapy until people get to know who you are. I don't know if you could call it prejudice, but there is a sense that they know who the right person is for a particular job. The person I replaced had been one of the Grosse Pointe people. I showed up with my tweed skirt, my jewel neck sweater and my string of pearls and looked the part.

It turned out I was given the position and worked with emotionally disturbed children. I met Eli Rubin, who was one of my mentors, and co-author on books and papers. (Llorens/Peters oral history, April 25–26, 2003, lines 721–767)

Llorens, working in a multidisciplinary team which included psychologist Rubin, discovered that 75% of the mentally ill children had cognitive-perceptual-motor dysfunction (Llorens, Levy, & Rubin, 1964). Llorens (1968b) conducted an exploratory study, to determine whether the perceptual motor dysfunction syndrome that Ayres studied in school children could be found in mentally ill children. Llorens' work led to knowing and becoming career-long friends with Ayres.

While working at the Lafayette Clinic, Llorens earned her Master of Arts in Vocational Rehabilitation from Wayne State University in 1962, and her Doctor of Philosophy in Education and Occupational Therapy from Walden University in 1976. She studied vocational rehabilitation in the late 1950s and early 1960s as did community member Stattel in the 1940s. Llorens shared her thinking: "The vocational rehabilitation program that I went in gave me a little bit of insurance in case we moved someplace where I needed a position that I wasn't able to get in occupational therapy." (Llorens/Peters oral history, April 25–26, 2003, lines 2998–3005).

Following her years at the Lafayette Clinic, working directly with West, Llorens accepted a Maternal and Child Health (MCH) Service, United States Department of Health, Education and Welfare (HEW) funded position as occupational therapy consultant, Comprehensive Child Care Project at Mount Zion Hospital in San Francisco from 1968 until 1971. In her community-based work with at risk families living in San Francisco's Western Addition housing projects, she demonstrated a new direction for occupational therapy practice. It was during this period that she participated in a White House Conference on Children and Youth, and received her Slagle lectureship. After 20 years of practicing occupational therapy, Llorens looked for a full-time teaching position, as well as a doctoral education program. Community member Alice Jantzen recruited Llorens to the University of Florida in 1971. Aware that they were moving to the South in 1971, the Llorens family contemplated potential racial tensions. She explained:

A small college town seemed to fit what we were looking for then. Alice (Jantzen) was very creative in her recruiting, because it was the South.

She made appointments for us to meet with the priest at St. Augustine Church, the Mayor of Gainesville who was black at the time, and other people in the community. However, there were incidences. Like Shands Teaching Hospital, where the occupational therapy program was located, had many bathrooms because it was built at the time where there were colored and white bathrooms. And there was a mini riot in Gainesville, and a brick was thrown into my husband's car. I still have the brick. Also, I could go any place in Gainesville I wanted between 8 a.m. and 5 p.m., because they might think I was the maid. But after 5 p.m. they might think I did not belong in that place. (Llorens/Peters oral history, April 25–26, 2003, lines 2067–2160)

Prior to leaving California, while Llorens was working at Mt. Zion Hospital and Medical Center, she started a doctoral program in educational psychology at the University of the Pacific. Community member Yerxa, while earning her doctorate at Boston University in the 1960s, spoke about learning a traditional science model during her educational psychology doctoral studies. Llorens, already an experienced clinical researcher for 10 years, shared her concerns about the educational psychology program at the University of the Pacific, recalling:

I enrolled in a traditional doctorate program at the University of the Pacific in educational psychology. The emphasis was on learning disability and that appealed to me at first, but I discovered traditional doctoral programs were looking for people they could mentor into their field. I really wasn't interested in becoming something other than an occupational therapist. I dropped out; for the first time in my life, I was mortified. (Llorens/Peters, April 25–26, 2003, lines 3,033–3,052)

Finding a non-traditional doctoral program at Walden University, Llorens and her husband, an educator, spent summers working on their doctoral degrees, while raising their daughter. Llorens retired as Professor Emeritus, San Jose State University, California where she was associate academic vice president of faculty affairs, from 1993 to 1996. Reflecting about her working past, she said:

It's interesting how if you live long enough, you have a career. Whereas, when I started out, I had a job. That's all I wanted, to pay my bills and take care of myself and other people. I still like that aspect of occupational therapy; it is a people-oriented profession. (Llorens/Peters oral history, April 25–26, 2003, lines 5,837–5,845)

Born during the depression years in 1933, Llorens, like community members Crampton, Cromwell, Gilfoyle, Stattel, Wiemer, and Yerxa, entered occupational therapy looking for a job to help people. Coming from humble roots, raised by her father and grandmother, Llorens first lived in Shreveport,

Louisiana. Like other community members, Llorens was close to her father. In 1943, her father moved the family to Detroit, Michigan, seeking better educational opportunities for his two daughters. Remembering her early years, Llorens said:

> We would be considered in the lower economic brackets. My dad was working at the post office in Shreveport. The values that we grew up with were more akin to middle or upper middle class. We knew etiquette and were given Emily Post books. We lived in a community where people knew each other, took care of each other's kids, like a village. There were women in our immediate community in Louisiana who were homemaker mentors. I learned vocational skills from them like canning and cooking. My grandmother was a housekeeper for a rich family. I learned how to cook from my grandmother, foods she made for the people she worked for, like English biscuits and tomato aspic. It was a segregated system, and I went to a segregated school. Education was the way to make it in the world. (Llorens/Peters oral history, lines 35–39, 10–14, 5,125–5,139, 218–228)

Llorens remembered her initial thoughts about entering college:

> I didn't know how I was going to be able to afford college. I figured if I had to I would go into the WACS, the Women Army Corps, and go to school like the GIs. It turned out my dad paid for it. (Llorens/Peters oral history, April 25–26, 2003, lines 248–260)

Starting her studies at the University of Puget Sound, Llorens was interested in the occupational therapy curriculum, while not quite understanding the profession. She explained:

> The curriculum was half science and half arts and crafts. I did well in the sciences at school. It was a nice combination. I learned to knit on two pencils with a string when I was 5 or 6 years old. My grandmother gave me weaving sets and wood burning sets at Christmas. I didn't know what occupational therapists did as a profession, but the curriculum was appealing. (Llorens/Peters oral history, April 25–26, 2003, lines 59–79)

Marrying after her college graduation, Llorens balanced a career and family. Llorens, raised a daughter, like Fidler and Gilfoyle, credited a supportive spouse who relocated for her career. She talked about her family life, recalling:

> I felt I could manage education, research, teaching, and practice, with a family. I could balance being a wife and mother but I couldn't do it if Joe hadn't been the kind of husband that he is, and the kind of father that he is. He shared the responsibilities for everything. I was established in my

career before he was.[40] The mobility was facilitated by my career. I don't think art teaching would have permitted him to have the kind of career that I had under any circumstances because my profession is predominantly a women's profession. (Llorens/Peters oral history, April 25–26, 2003, lines 1,270–1,272; 3,759–3,793)

Balancing a full life and career, Llorens forged new professional territory. When asked if she saw herself more as a scholar or as a leader she responded:

I ideally see myself as an occupational therapist who had the opportunity to be an educator, clinician, an academician, researcher, and consultant. But my basic identity is that of an occupational therapy practitioner. I would never give up occupational therapy because that has permitted me to do the other things that I have done. It provided me the opportunities to live out my dream, or my father's dream.

He was proud of the fact that I never lost my identity of who I am, that I could move back and forth between cultures. African Americans of my generation know a lot more about white culture then whites of that same generation know about African American culture. I've always known that I was first colored, then I was Negro, then I was black and African American. But I've always been me. My dad raised us both to believe that we could do anything we wanted to do. We were not restrained by the fact that we were women or that we were African American.(Llorens/Peters oral history, April 25–26, 2003, lines 5,775–5,793; 5,064–5,071; 2,508–2,518; 4,972–4,988)

Llorens, an occupational therapy insider and sustainer, broadened and diversified the occupational therapy profession. Like Bing, who experienced being the first and only male AOTA president, Llorens broke new ground.

This section discussed eight occupational therapy leaders and scholars who were members of the community of therapists. Therapists Cromwell, Gilfoyle, and Wiemer, each contributing to occupational therapy's knowledge base, made political strides, showing that knowledge development and politics can mix. Therapists Crampton, Stattel and Welles represented the community's old-guard supporters and sustainers. Working well with political movers, they also kept the community "sisterhood" spirit alive, maintaining insider and outsider connections. For example Welles' spoke easily about her career-long friendship with outsider Reilly, and Crampton recalled working with Mosey in the 1960s. Therapists Bing and Llorens contributed to occupational therapy knowledge while challenging old traditions, and led AOTA and AOTF when scholarship was a priority. The next section discusses the move to science, and explores the nature of occupational therapy knowledge.

SECTION VI: THE DILEMMA OF PHILOSOPHY AND SCIENCE

How did a small group of occupational therapy scholars and leaders who had different viewpoints, dodge potential rifts to move occupational therapy towards a science-based profession? Secondly, how did science fit into a philosophically based practice profession? This section explores the dilemma of how members in the community separated in their thinking about occupational therapy's knowledge base. Although there were differences, a full debate amongst therapists leading to dissonance wasn't prevalent in the occupational therapy culture. The community insiders politically chartered AOTA and AOTF direction. Dissonant views were noted and camps were quietly aligned, with insiders supporting a predominantly philosophical knowledge base and outsiders or futurists supporting a scientific knowledge base. The community of therapists remained unclear about whether occupational therapy is an art (philosophy) or a science, because they spoke about both interchangeably. Based on this study, however, those interviewed spoke more about a philosophical rather than scientific base, even when they were using terms like theoretical foundations and research. This lack of clarity is discussed later in this section while identifying milestones, like the development of AOTF, and the community culture and mindset that prevailed. Finally, in this section the author presents an analysis and interpretation of how discussions about philosophy and science furthered knowledge development and professionalization in the larger "System of Profession," including moving through system disturbances that brought about change.

Philosophy or Science: A System Disturbance

The philosophy and science dilemma in occupational therapy is an internal system disturbance between community insiders (political movers and sustainers), and outsiders (theorists and futurists). Community insiders, supporting a philosophical approach, and outsiders, supporting a scientific approach to practice, sought mutual avenues to explain occupational therapy's contribution to society. Occupational therapy's philosophical base included professional beliefs, ethics, the art of practice and science.[41] Occupational therapy's science-based body of knowledge included theories or theoretical postulates, and the methods of science, including observing physical phenomena, formulating questions, investigating findings, and drawing conclusions (Mosey, 1996).

The profession gradually moved away from a 30-year tradition where practice was based on philosophical beliefs to more systematic methodologies and empirical studies. Seeking scientific rationales for questions, those therapists supporting a more scientific approach to practice were in the minority amongst a community of therapists who either mislabeled philosophy as scientific or had no interest in changing traditional occupational therapy views. This was evident in confusing discussions about the nature of occupational therapy philosophy and science pertaining to theory development and research.

Community members weighed both sides, identifying occupational therapy's scientific and/or philosophic knowledge base. Were they the same or different, and how did they apply to occupational therapy practice or professional development? Debate and discourse didn't come easily to therapists, as Yerxa explained:

> I think we're all very nice people and we haven't liked conflict. I don't think we were far enough developed to be able to conceptualize enough to debate. In order to debate I think you have to have the ability to put things into the conceptual realm. We still had a hands-on idea. The sciences were borrowed from other fields. It was more like, how do you do it rather than should it be done this way; it's quite striking. (Yerxa/Peters oral history, April 21–22, 2003, lines 2,908–2,920)

Llorens echoed Yerxa's thoughts about community members' process in discussing occupational therapy's knowledge base. Stylistically, the community did not confront each other or criticize readily. Speaking about her experiences chairing AOTF's Research Advisory Council, a group consisting of occupational therapy's most notable contributors, Llorens stated:

> I don't know if there was much discourse about direction, particularly in the Research Advisory Council. That was a compatible group. Among the theory group, each person was identified for his or her own work. In general there was an attempt to try to bring some of that together. I don't think it happened. There was a lot of discussion, and I think some acrimony. Actually, there hasn't been enough of the kind of discourse that allows us to battle it out. (Llorens/Peters oral history, April 25–26, 2003, lines 5,661–5,694)

Perhaps at the heart of the discussion is how did an evolving science fit into a philosophically-rooted profession? Old-guard insiders would deny any fit, new-guard sustainers and political movers may see the change as eventual, and theorists would argue that science was imperative. I argue that in spite of the traditional stronghold that the philosophical viewpoint commanded, science was a move to professional survival, particularly amongst other allied health care professions in the 1960s and 1970s. Otherwise, occupational therapy would have remained too small, obsolete, and undiscovered to remain viable. Occupational therapy grew because it became more like medicine, or scientific in the 1960s and 1970s, allowing it to stand on its own merits and body of knowledge rather than in the shadow of medicine, as in the 1950s. For example, Gilfolye rebuked medicine's 1960s reductionistic focus, saying it didn't fit occupational therapy's philosophically-grounded caring. (Gilfoyle/Peters oral history, February 10–11, 2003, lines 2,482–2,487)

Therapists in the 1970s were able to answer their own questions about why what they did worked based on empirical evidence. Fidler, for one, didn't see a move toward science occurring. She questioned, and more pointedly she debated, the thesis that occupational therapy evolved to a science based profession between 1950 and 1980. Fidler spiritedly argued:

> No it's a misnomer. What the move was, was to provide a rationale for what we were doing. That was seen in all probability as scientific, but that doesn't make it science. Medicine is a science because they have researched and found evidence to address their questions.
>
> The process that we went through was hardly scientific. Somebody had an idea that this is what happened, or I said I know I practiced this and had seen these results for these years.[42] But there was no bona fide research or investigation that explored and raised more questions about what needed to happen or was happening.
>
> If we were really scientific, we would ask questions, and each question you ask would raise other questions. The pursuit of the question, not the answer, is the process that enables growth, knowledge, and understanding. (Fidler/Peters oral history, March 6–7, 2003, lines 7,102–7,114; 601–613; 624–634)

Given Fidler's argument, research methodology was rudimentary in the 1950s, and developed sophistication in the late 1960s and 1970s as more therapists sought graduate education. A science mindset and enculturation, however, was emergent in the 1950s, though not widely identified. Ironically, Fidler, early on, argued and educated therapists about the importance of theoretical thinking. She identified herself and challenged others to ask questions about occupational therapy's efficacy and uniqueness. She also mentored Mosey, who supported the thesis, and facilitated occupational therapy to a science-based profession. Agreeing with Mosey and disagreeing with Fidler's stance, occupational therapy theory was supporting a scientific foundation to practice. Fidler's and Rood's theoretical work was prominent in 1950s, followed by Ayres, Mosey, and Reilly in the 1960s and 1970s. The issue and core of the dilemma is that Fidler, like other insiders didn't identify occupational therapy as scientific, but rather philosophical in nature. Fidler stated:

> There still is very little scientific inquiry in OT. We adapted, we took on scientific statements and credibility that belonged to medicine, but not our own. But a pure science base is too narrow, because there is a philosophy. A science base does not acknowledge the symbolic nature of culture down through the ages. I'm not certain that OT should be a science. We have a philosophical base most certainly, most certainly. (Fidler/Peters oral history, March 6–7, 2003, lines 6,862–6,873; 6,797–6,798; 6,996–7,006)

What appears most evident in these community discussions, including Fidler's critique, is that theory and philosophy were intertwined. Llorens talked about how she mixed philosophy and theory in her Slagle lecture, stating:

> My Slagle lecture combined some philosophy and theory. Facilitating growth and development is really the theory. The philosophy is more related to a developmental orientation, or a human growth and human development orientation in terms of philosophy. (Llorens/Peters oral history, April 25–26, 2003, lines 2,804–2,811)

Gilfoyle also saw a bridge between occupational therapy philosophy, theory, and occupation. She stated:

> We do proclaim that we have a philosophic base; that is what we value. With that we also recognize the importance of theory, and that theory and our premises will be dynamic forever. The philosophy of occupational therapy is going to emerge, and it will grow because we will have ways of demonstrating what it is that we do that makes a difference. That's why we do research; it's not that we want to be science based, it is to build our philosophy. I think the way to become science-based is to define your philosophy. We are not, and we're not going to emerge as a science. I wouldn't want us to. I think philosophy combines science and art beautifully. (Gilfoyle/Peters oral history, February 10–11, 2003, lines 3,121–3,150; 2,610–2,624; 2,654–2,663; 2,673–2,679; 2,447–2,463; 2,554–2,556; 1,682–1,683)

Talking about occupational therapy as an art and science, Cromwell points back to the arts and crafts "doing" foundation of the field, seeing the profession strongly grounded in a philosophical base. Cromwell explained:

> You can't lose the roots from which we stem, which was arts and crafts and doing activities with hands. Our theory base comes from that kind of doing. It's a science to the extent that we want to measure. I hope we don't fall into the trap of trying to be so scientific that we're just being nuts and bolts people. I think times dictate that we have to prove this happened or could happen. To that extent they may call us science. But I think we're more a humanistic profession, because it's the ways in which we involve people in solving their own problems that are the deep things about OT. (Cromwell/Peters oral history, April 28–29, 2003, lines 7,352–7,393)

If science wasn't discussed using the label, it was addressed in terms of functional activities or therapeutic occupation. This change paralleled historical events where occupational therapists work and role expanded, like meeting soldiers needs following World War II. According to West, "functional activities came around World War II to distinguish them from diversion" (Bing, 1982, Slagle meeting notes, private papers). Although there was a shift to identify occupation and activities as functional, or scientific, there was also a belief that they were philosophically rooted, or labeled as both. Wiemer explained:

> I wish to distinguish activities and occupation. Occupation returns to occupational therapy roots and undergirds professionalism. When I came aboard as president, there still was so much pure entertainment going on in the name of OT. (Wiemer/Peters oral history, March 18–19, 2003, lines 2,901–2,943)

Along these lines, Gilfoyle stated:

> When I left school, I had a belief system, not a theory about the use of crafts and occupation. But it was certainly the beginnings of a theory because you have to begin with what you believe in and its value. (Gilfoyle/Peters oral history, February 10–11, 2003, lines 192–204)

The term occupation, identified philosophically and scientifically, is similar to other abstract concepts. Without specific definition it leads to misinterpretation. Fidler weighed in best, stating:

> Its like that damn term occupation, it drives me up the wall! We're all supposed to know what it means when it means different things to different people, and they contradict one another. How can you decide about something that complex that is ubiquitous in our discipline without research? We define things by asking a committee or a so-called leader to define it, and what they say is gospel. (Fidler/Peters oral history, March 6–7, 2003, lines 4,210–4,221)

Because of the possibility of misinterpretation, Yerxa believed that defining what type of science one is discussing is important, because most peoples—occupational therapists—view, was that of traditional science (Yerxa/Peters oral history, lines 4,052–4,054). Imbedded in the following passage, Yerxa spoke about science and philosophy when she interpreted Reilly's theoretical work, thus illustrating another crossover, and how in her opinion occupational therapy philosophy was scientifically grounded. In Yerxa's view, Reilly stood apart and didn't support traditional science at a time when it was prevalent, stating:

> Mary Reilly was a visionary. When other people talked about that (traditional science), she was talking about systems, environments, and how important interests were in human motivation. She never lost her belief, as I see her work. She never lost her belief in the significance of the human engaging in activity. She had an incredible grounding in OT (occupational therapy) and in Adolf Meyer. I don't think most people understood what she was saying; it's too bad because she did have

brilliant ideas. She's very philosophical, and was talking about the move away from positivism and reductionism practically out of the gate. I think she's the first person I saw use the word epistemology in the literature. (Yerxa/Peters oral history, April 21–22, 2003, lines 3,809–3,817; 3,899–3,910; 3,886–3,895)

This section discussed a system disturbance between philosophy and science, including an analysis of occupational therapy knowledge development from 1950 until 1980. Community insiders argued that occupational therapy's knowledge was philosophically based. Community outsiders supported a scientific knowledge base. When community insiders spoke about a science-based knowledge, theory development, and research, and when their words were deconstructed, one discovered that they spoke more about philosophy than science. This established a pattern in occupational therapy of mislabeling and not defining key concepts that remains today. The next section will discuss occupational therapy theory development and research.

Theory Development: Science and Philosophy Confusion

Occupational therapy theory originated from other disciplines. Initially physicians and psychologists shared their frames of reference. Llorens, talked about conceptualizing her 1969 Slagle lecture, recalling:

> The theorists that informed my Eleanor Clarke Slagle lecture and had the most meaning to me were Gesell, Erikson, and Piaget. The notion that activity could bring about change in behavior, could unstick a dysfunctional development, came from the first definition of occupation therapy that I learned, which is occupational therapy is any activity, mental or physical, etc. in Willard and Spackman.[43] (Llorens/Peters oral history, April 25–26, 2003, lines 6,474–6,524)

Yerxa, however, believed that as occupational therapy theoretical knowledge developed, there was a break from medicine's pathology model. In her view, "if we hadn't severed from medicine, we would always be constrained, we would never achieve professionalism, or the ability to contribute to society the way we did" (Yerxa/Peters, line 2,701–2,705). This break came with some community resistance, for example the American Medical Association maintained influence accrediting occupational therapy educational programs, therefore curriculum was complimentary to the medical model. For example Yerxa remembered neurological theoretical treatment approaches that she taught at the College of Puget Sound, now the University of Puget Sound, in 1955 and 1956, saying:

> The popular theorists in physical disabilities, the NDT (neurodevelopmental treatment) and Kaiser approaches; Kabot, Signe Brunstromm,

and Rood to bring about a response by using sensory input. They used those techniques with polio patients. That's how Jean Ayres started. She was working at Kabat Kaiser and using mass patterns to try to bring about a better neurological response recruiting more impulses for people who had polio. (Yerxa/Peters oral history, April 21–22, 2003, lines 1,244–1,283)

Psychoanalytic theory dominated mental health occupational therapy in the 1950s and 1960s. A case in point, Bing remembered a workshop at Nebraska Psychiatric Institute coordinated by occupational therapist Dwyer Dundon, a Bing and Fidler colleague, that illustrates psychoanalytic theory's dominance over developmental theoretical frameworks in occupational therapy. He stated:

> The two day workshop at Nebraska Psychiatric Institute had doctors Hasan, a psychiatrist and psychoanalyst, and Fern Azima, a lay psychoanalyst, making some headway into OT (occupational therapy) as gurus. The first day was given to psychoanalytical thought and its implications for OT. I was the keynote speaker the second day, and spoke about the theories of Erik Erikson, Carl Rogers, Karen Horney, and Erich Fromm. I said we had an obligation to know the prevailing theories in psychiatric practice and develop a rational synthesis that supports our treatment contentions. Fern came over to me in a sicky sweet snide way, and said I would not last long in OT unless I came over to her side. She pointed out that Gail Fidler was much more influential and deserved our undivided attention.[44] (Bing/Peters oral history, February 21, 2003, lines 504–526)

Workshops proved to be where therapists talked about knowledge development. West's talent at obtaining grants helped gather and create occupational therapy's "think tank." One example is the National Institute of Mental Health grant-funded project that began in 1954. Resulting in *Psychiatric Occupational Therapy*, edited by West, a 1959 AOTA publication summarizing the Allenberry Inn Conference, Boiling Springs, Pennsylvania, November 13–19, 1956.[45] Gail Fidler coordinated the project, working with West and committee chair Elizabeth Ridgway, and Marion Crampton, an executive committee member. The project's goal was to "examine, assess and define the current concepts and practice of occupational therapy in psychiatry" (West, 1959, p. xi) Harry Solomon, MD, a Massachusetts psychiatrist whom Crampton worked with, introduced the text, stating that there was:

> an inspired renaissance of thinking about the place of occupational therapy and the professional requirements of the trained worker. The present drive is for a more scientific approach, at least an understanding of the principles for the development of the therapeutic relationship . . . In

reading the material one is made aware that the occupational therapist of today has a high motivation for developing a distinctly professional status. (p. iv)

Although it was considered complementary when written, Solomon's introduction skirted the issue of occupational therapy's autonomy as a bona fide scientific profession. Rather he acknowledged therapists motivation, supporting the argument that if occupational therapy was more like medicine, then it would evolve as a science-based profession. Crampton thought about Solomon's perception that occupational therapy was evolving and developing a more scientific approach. Crampton stated:

I don't think that was in my head. I knew things were changing, but I probably wouldn't have described it like that. That was when we were moving into psychotherapy and psychoanalysis, which was quite different from descriptive psychiatry. At the time I became supervisor of OT for the Department of Mental Health, I felt OT was moving, and I was more with the descriptive psychiatry. I felt I didn't have the knowledge that I should have, and by going to conferences I learned. (Crampton/Peters oral history, March 1, 2003, lines1,796–1,799; 1,624–1,631; 1,240–1,247)

Crampton's response captures an occupational therapy crossroads, when description and an intuitive knowing, familiar and grounded in practice, was not enough. Yerxa (1991), writing about occupational therapy knowing and epistemology stated "To be true to our patients, ourselves, and our ethical traditions, we as occupational therapists need to seek or invent new ways of knowing" (p. 200).

Identifying this challenge in the 1950s, Crampton knew that treatment needed theoretical grounding. Yerxa, characterizing a 1950s occupational therapy, described learning a descriptive or "how-to" approach rather than a theoretical focus when she was a student at the University of Southern California. She explained:

When I was a student it was a 'how-to' approach and activity analysis. This is how you treat somebody with these symptoms. It was all by diagnosis like schizophrenia and manic depression. The same with polio, the muscle test was the Rosetta stone. It sat well with our aspirations to become like medicine. You know it's very much the medical model, diagnostic, treatment, and cure approach.

We had these two streams dichotomized between psychiatry and physical disabilities. With physical disabilities you used Willard and Spackman, Clare Spackman's work, and the bicycle saw.[46] I think if I ever heard the word theory, it was Freudian psychiatry and the Fidlers' use of activity for psychodynamic purposes. (Yerxa/Peters oral history, April 21–22, 2003, lines1,290–1,311; 1,321–1,340)

Fidler talked about developing the psychoanalytically based theory that Yerxa remembered in the 1950s. Fidler's projective theoretical work began in the 1940s and evolved to her Lifestyle Performance Model (Fidler & Velde, 1999; Fidler, 1964, 1969, 1983, 1994, 1997). As a young therapist in the late 1940s, Fidler met Sidney Licht, MD,[47] who suggested she begin formalizing her innovative thinking and writing her ideas. She remembered those post-World War II conversations, saying:

> I didn't know what a theory was, and at that point I couldn't have cared less; it was never in my head. What I was interested in was exploring the many questions I had about activities and how they were related to human behavior. I was obsessed and continue to be. A theory evolved and it's taken me a lifetime.
>
> I became convinced empirically that a relationship existed between the kind of person and the kind of activity, and that activities had meaning in and of themselves. It took me time to convince myself that I had a valid hypothesis. I struggled years thinking about the meaning of activities, and how does this relate to living.
>
> One weekend I went home to visit my parents; they lived in a little house at the edge of the woods with dirt paths. I walked through the woods thinking and suddenly it was like a light went on in my head. I said I'm making this too difficult, and it's about enabling survival with some sense of satisfaction. (Fidler/Peters oral history, March 6–7, 2003, lines 4,847–4,890; 6,479–6,564)

Other community members introduced and applied developmental and behavioral theories to occupational therapy. Theorists like Ayres, Reilly, Fidler, and Mosey developed frames of reference that connected theory and practice, most notably in the 1960s and 1970s. Broadening the profession's science base, Ayres (1963) and Llorens (1968b) for example, studied children with cognitive-perceptual-motor dysfunction, thus applying their frames of reference to clinical research. Yerxa believed that Reilly's *Occupational Behavior* and Ayres *Sensory Integration* frames of references are two examples in occupational therapy literature. She explained:

> If you read *Occupational Behavior*, it's not about pathology, it's about how significant people's occupational behavior is to their adaptation to their environments. Both Reilly and Ayres created theories that were basic and not applied. They asked the question: what is there about human beings that we look at in a unique way; that we need to understand? Ultimately, it would be scientifically tested. But they developed basic theories about human beings that would then enable them to be applied. They moved the profession forward in a completely different way. (Yerxa/Peters oral history, April 21–22, 2003, lines 4,216–4,262)

Yerxa's idea that Reilly and Ayres developed basic occupational therapy theories differs from Mosey's (1995) taxonomy and explanation of applied scientific inquiry. I agree with Mosey, seeing occupational therapy's frames of reference as guidelines for practice, namely applied, rather than basic theoretical information. In that view, Ayres' sensory integration frames of reference apply theoretical information to answer questions arising from clinical problems.

Llorens captured the discussions that summarized occupational therapy's theoretical development in the 1960s and 1970s, seeing it as internal regional camps. She stated:

> The domain of concern of occupational therapy, or what we really should be concerning ourselves with, and the language that people were using was discussed. Anne Mosey was using 'domain' and I don't think that the people on the West Coast were using that language at all. There were these definite divisions that had to do with language. Occupational behavior belonged to Reilly, and other people who didn't feel comfortable with that had other terms they used. 'Domain of concern' was one of those phrases. I didn't have a camp, and I was probably seen as more objective. I believed in a developmental frame of reference, and I think that Willie (West) did as well. (Llorens/Peters oral history, April 25–26, 2003, lines 4,289–4,323)

Newly prepared with unique occupational therapy frames of reference, occupational therapy scholars and leaders entered clinical and academic settings. This shift did not readily filter to the larger membership in the 1950s, when practice was based upon apprentice training, or through a trial-and-error process. Ideally, 1960s and 1970s occupational therapists would have utilized theoretical information, however, practice shifted slowly. Perhaps therapists in the larger membership did not understand the significance of theory in practice. West contemplated this very issue, knowing the merits of theory development and research. There was a chasm separating the community of therapists' more esoteric concerns like knowledge development, and gaining research funding, compared to the larger membership's daily responsibilities, including keeping pace with patient load, physician's requests and staffing deficits.

This tug between the need to develop a theoretical basis for practice and the demands that the larger membership addressed in daily practice coincided with sociologists' and historians' debates about the place of expert knowledge in practice-based professions like medicine (Fidler, 1979b; Friedson, 1984). How was theory going to be understood and utilized in everyday practice? As stated in Section I, a unique body of occupational therapy knowledge alone was not enough to make occupational therapy viable in a competitive health care environment. Knowledge was an important conceptual underpinning, but not a catchall for the profession. I argue that expansion and change to a science-based profession was not an outgrowth of intellectual elitism over the populist membership, as Colman (1984) characterized the division among therapist. Occupational therapy scholars were few in numbers and community outsiders stayed on the community's fringe, either by choice or exclusion. Rather, community insiders like West, Fidler, Cromwell, and Wiemer, who were politically astute, and who assessed health care trends, knew the timing was right to move toward science. They were occupational therapy's agents who sought and gained federal research money that moved occupational therapy into a different playing field. Political insiders and old-guard sustainers gained the resources to support the theorists beyond their own funding, to develop the professional knowledge that better served society.

Occupational therapy, a predominantly female profession, functioning at the baccalaureate level, had hurdles to cross prior to making any significant strides. West, discovering solutions, found the talented therapists and created environments for them to engage in the experiments that supported practice. It wasn't until the late 1970s that occupational therapists started making noticeable strides toward theory development. This was partly due to the small cadre of graduate-level therapists, and partly due to the predominant belief system that a philosophical foundation best supported practice. The next section will discuss how research developed, swaying the philosophy and science pendulum toward science.

Research Development: A Shift Toward Science

Few occupational therapists were engaging in research in the 1950s and 1960s. Ayres (1955a, 1955b, 1955c), an exception, presented her research findings in the 1950s. Such voids in research can be linked to education level, a limited number of occupational therapists able to mentor such efforts, geographic isolation, and few collaboration opportunities. Yerxa (1981), giving insight to the 1970s decade, discussed occupational therapy's research status. She stated, "occupational therapy research is delimited necessarily by the stages of development of occupational therapy theory," (p. 821). Why did it take more than 20 years to start seeing some national-level membership support that promoted research? One reason may be that some therapists considered knowledge development an academic exercise, and one that was not part of the "real" world. Llorens remembered occupational therapy's 1960s and 1970s landscape, saying "I think that some practicing therapists thought theory wasn't connected to practice in the 1960s and 1970s, that it was pie in the sky. I think that some therapists still feel that there really isn't a need for theory." (Llorens/ Peters oral history, April 25–26, 2003, lines 2,769–2,782; 4,549–4,573)

Compounding this, Llorens said:

Acceptance was the driving force, because most practitioners thought research was driven by academia because those were the people who were gaining in research or needed to publish. There weren't a lot of therapists in research in the 1960s. I didn't know enough to know in those days that I was considered an exception or doing something different. I truly believed that's what we should be doing. (Llorens/Peters oral history, April 25–26, 2003, lines 4,549–4,573)

AOTA had early research concerns, including forming the scientific study and research committee in 1946, chaired by Lucy G. Morse of Massachusetts General Hospital, who submitted a May 1946 report summarizing "Bedside Projects for Men" that involved task assemblage (AOTA Archives, Collection RG 4, Box NR 53, File NR 375). Upon expanding in 1949, the committee on research and application was chaired by Margaret S. Rood and included members Sr. Jeanne Marie [Bonnet] and Myra McDaniel. The committee's October 1950 year-end report noted research collaboration between St. Catherine's College and the Hines Veterans Administration Hospital. The committee gathered resources like those therapists with master's degrees and research funding sources to be explored, including the Kellogg Foundation, Upjohn Medical House, the National Society for Crippled Children and Adults, Inc., National Mental Health Act Funds, and the National Foundation for Infantile Paralysis (AOTA Archives, Coll RG 4, Box NR 53, File NR 375).

Adding to this, therapists like Fidler and Gilfoyle lacked research knowledge and the experience one gains while pursuing graduate education and doctoral studies. Occupational therapy lacked advanced educational programs. It wasn't until the 1970s, at New York University, that the first occupational therapy doctoral program was established. Research was not consistently grounded in theory in the 1950s and 1960s. I question whether these quasi-experimental exercises that therapists labeled research or clinical investigations were incomplete studies based on trial and error or traditional means, or "the way things were done."

Investigations described phenomena, or testing procedures, or equipment design and use, but lacked conceptual frameworks to ground comprehensive studies. For example, Stattel remembered her data-gathering experiences at Kessler Institute in New Jersey from 1950 until 1956. Stattel, a baccalaureate-level therapist in the 1950s, used this Kessler work as inspiration for her Slagle lecture, stating:

Research always came comfortably. When I was at Kessler, we were testing, we had weights tied to patient's hands, but it was not formal research as we know it today. If I wanted to find something out, I would put up a pulley or I would set up a metronome. I designed equipment, like removable bars that screwed in and out on standing tables or I would put on wheels. I never published it; I never had time to publish. You had to make tests to see what results would promote OT. I said to Dr. Kessler if you want before-and-after pictures of cases, I'd take them. We can start on patients where we know we can see results. (Stattel/Peters oral history, November 21, 1997, lines 591–612)

Mental health, one of the first practice areas to utilize a theoretical framework, based on Fidler's interpretation of psychoanalytic theory as it applied to occupational therapy in the 1950s, lacked studies. Fidler spoke about mental health research in the 1950s and 1960s (Fidler, 1958, 1964, 1966a, 1966b) illustrating a void in that practice area by saying:

> I was always concerned about research. In the 1950s we had nothing; it was anecdotal. I don't know any research in terms of mental health or the psychological aspects of OT. Well, I think the proof in the pudding is by the 1970s we didn't exist. It was part of a total picture. I don't think we died off simply because we weren't ready to cope with that. I think psychiatry died off by the mid-70 s. (Fidler/Peters oral history, March 6–7, 2003, lines 7,041–7,079)

If research did occur in mental health, it didn't make it to publication. For example Bing remembered a thwarted research effort with a psychologist, recalling:

> In 1956, I hooked up with a member of the psychology division at Norwich State Hospital in Connecticut. We set out to do a study of chronic women patients using the newly developed thorazine for one group and occupational therapy for this group, then occupational therapy for a non-thorazine group. We were interested in finding out what effect the drug had on following directions, accomplishing simple to complex tasks, particularly in crafts. I handed my share of the work over to the psychologist. I never heard what happened but I suspect he ditched the whole thing. (Bing/Peters oral history, February 22, 2003, lines 660–675)

Lacking in most of these early research attempts, few therapists spoke about collaboration with other professionals who did have research experience and training like psychologists. Llorens, for example was an exception, who unlike Bing, successfully collaborated and co-published with psychologist Rubin in the 1960s. She claimed this collaborative work went beyond an exchange of ideas, but also served as training, and mentorship. The larger problem pointed to a lack of research enculturation, or research mindedness. Fidler saw this problem stemming from occupational therapy education and gender characteristics (Fidler, 1979a). This was a point well taken, considering the 1950s and 1960s curriculum focused on craft and activity analysis, rather than research methodologies. Secondly, occupational therapy academic program directors continued recruiting conservative young women who had similar values and beliefs as their own. Fidler stated:

> If we had research that was reviewed in other science journals it would be a draw. But we don't do that kind of quality research. It's understandable that until such time as we do something about our education, that isn't going to happen. I think the other issue is the persons whom we

recruit. These are not persons who characteristically think logically, with a research orientation and attitude to life. They just are not the questioning people. They don't question, and that's part of being a woman. (Fidler/ Peters oral history, March 6–7, 2003, lines 4,087–4,097; 7,144–7,157)

Further illustrating 1960s research beginnings, Gilfoyle remembered her work at Craig Rehabilitation Institute and Children's Hospital in Denver from 1960 until 1965. Gilfoyle's early research interests, largely unfunded, stemmed from her own curiosities and were secondary to her daily practice demands. She stated:

It was early in my career when I began to ask some questions. I know I'm doing something, I can see it, but I can't tell somebody why. I was very intrigued because if a child with cerebral palsy could be helped by the stability of the leg brace, why couldn't a child with cerebral palsy be helped by the stability of a hand brace? So I went over to Children's hospital and did some consulting work to fit children with cerebral palsy with hand braces. (Gilfoyle/Peters oral history, February 10–11, 2003, lines 213–220, 430–477)

In spite of AOTAs early organizing attempts, including AOTA's Research and Special Projects Committee 1962 report suggesting AOTF handle the association's research needs, West identified a continued research void (AOTA archives, Collection RG 4, Box NR 53, File NR 375). West was concerned and believed that occupational therapy lacked a national membership commitment to support needed research in 1976 (Llorens & Snyder, 1987).

Another concern addressed occupational therapists' not meeting a certain type of research standard or ideal that supported the stance that basic scientists were "real" scientists. Welles, referring to this paradigm, thought basic science was beyond occupational therapy's scope. She explained:

I had some papers published, but I didn't do much research. Some physicians were scientists, like Dr. Millikan, a great friend of the family. Dr. Robert A. Millikan is the man who discovered the electron. He was a friend of my father's and was on the board at the hospital where I taught. I'd see him often, and we would say hello. (Welles/Peters oral history, April 28–29, 2003, lines 3,647–3,662)

Adding to the complexities about research type, Gilfoyle and Yerxa spoke about expanding occupational therapy's methodology, including both basic and applied scientific research. Gilfoyle stated:

The research we needed had to be bench research because that's what we knew about research, the basic sciences. When I became aware of applied science, I began to think that that's the route we need to go. I think Mosey's *Frames of Reference* influenced me. We were developing the curriculum around related services in the public schools and began to see there was something beyond the medical model. We don't want to clone ourselves. We want to understand the basic sciences, and how they can be integrated and utilized to support the philosophy of the profession. (Gilfoyle/Peters oral history, February 10–11, 2003, lines 2,491–2,502; 2,516–2,545)

Gilfoyle's previous statement illustrated the belief that basic science supported the philosophy of the profession. This cross over between science and philosophy is one example of the interchange that therapists made between philosophy and science. Although both words were used, few defined how they viewed occupational therapy philosophy and science. This added to confusion about occupational therapy's direction amongst community members, with insiders holding philosophy in high regards, and others seeing science as a new direction.

Those community members, responding to 1960s and 1970s science trends, supported the idea that a science-based body of knowledge, that is, an accumulation of applied scientific information that guided practice would insure occupational therapy's authority and professional knowledge.[48-51]

West, and other community members like Llorens, Fidler, Gilfoyle, and Yerxa, became involved in AOTA and AOTF's Research Advisory Council created in 1979. The council's mission encouraged:

The development and testing of theory to provide evidence that supports or refutes hypotheses relative to the effectiveness of practice and must support research that contributes to the broadening of the knowledge base that is the mother lode for practice. (Llorens & Gillette, 1985, p. 143)

AOTF Executive Director Martha Kirkland remembers events leading to the advisory council development, stating:

In 1978, AOTA asked the foundation to take responsibility for research. I remember that most dramatically. There were definitely two sides of research. One side is clear, the scholarly work to understand your profession with ideas and theories. Then you need to test; you have to test how well those ideas can be applied to practice. Can you reliably use these ideas to construct an intervention that makes some tangible difference?

Secondly, there was a need in the profession for more people who could do research, and developing a series of scholars who work within a certain line of reasoning around some basic ideas. That meant we had to build capacities for standards. (Kirkland/Peters interview, March 21, 2003, lines 608–645)

Coming together, doing AOTA and AOTF committee work, conferences, or workshops, the community of therapists represented the profession's think tank. They addressed the nature of occupational therapy's knowledge.

They debated whether occupational therapy was a scientifically- or philosophically-based profession, boiling this debate down to a science and art discussion. Gilfoyle believed "the unique blending of the science of occupation and the art of our caring relationships distinguishes our profession. Science provides facts to guide practice and assure accountability for our services. But we must also value art as the dimension that creates the conditions for science to be used (1987a, p. 12)." Llorens discussed occupational therapy's conceptual foundation, and science's status, stating:

> Occupational therapy has aspects of art and aspects of science, but I don't think the science is well-articulated or understood. I'm aware of the people who felt that we did not have a scientific basis, and while neurophysiology, sociology, and behavioral sciences were the underpinnings for human development there was still this longing for a finite unique science of occupation. My belief is that still isn't going to be the case. (Llorens/Peters oral history, April 25–26, 2003, lines 5,491–5,494; 5,558–5,576)

This section discussed how occupational theory and research development shifted the philosophy and science pendulum toward science. Research in the 1950s and 1960s was informal, anecdota, and typically not theoretically grounded. By the late 1960s and 1970s, shifts were noted with more theoretical work present. Community members spoke about their research experiences and changing views. Although different, community members presented a blurring of occupational therapy philosophy and science. The next section will discuss how philosophy took precedence in occupational therapy, and continued blurring lines between philosophical and scientific knowledge.

The Philosophical Base Project: Sealed Records

Differing slightly, but also similar to today's scientific debate about basic and/or applied occupational therapy research discussed in Section I, the community of therapists deliberated the merits of a scientific and/or philosophical occupational therapy knowledge base. Yerxa (1974) presented and identified occupational therapy's "pre-scientific" research status, citing the following four reasons for her analysis:

> First, our value system as occupational therapy practitioners has often been centered upon the welfare of individuals, grounded in humanistic caring. We tend to view scientific research as 'hyperobjective, disinterested, and manipulative.'
>
> Second, when faced with the dilemma of giving time to serve people who need us or taking the time to plan and conduct research, the immediate people needs will frequently exert a stronger pull than the less immediate need to know.

Thirdly, we suffer from fragmentation of the conceptual framework and theoretical disassociation. Should occupational therapy be science based at all, or perhaps be artistic, intuitive or philosophic?

Fourth, the ability to perform research requires the development of considerable knowledge and skill. Few schools provide opportunities for either undergraduates or graduate students to gain sufficient knowledge and directed research experience. (pp. 676–677)

Capturing occupational therapy's pull between a philosophic humanist belief system and a more objective science, set the 1970s stage for occupational therapy's philosophy or science dilemma. Celebrating occupational therapy's 60th anniversary as a health care profession, discussions culminated in what grew into the 6.5-year AOTA "philosophical base project," starting April 1977 through AOTA's Commission on Practice and expanding to an ad hoc committee of various AOTA committee chairpersons and the executive board in June 1977.[52] Developing project strategies, this group cited the following from AOTA's Task Force on Social Issues (1974) paper justifying the project and ultimately the profession's survival:

Occupational therapy must begin more serious work in the development of accepted theoretical frames of reference, theories, standardized evaluations and treatment procedures, research, special studies and publication. Practice must be based on theory rather than being technique-oriented practice. (Bing, 1982, private papers, AOTA Philosophical Base Project, Agenda, p. 2)

I question whether this explanation better justified pursuing a scientific rather than a philosophical occupational therapy knowledge base. Mosey delineates philosophical assumptions from scientific statements. In her view, both are components of a profession's fundamental knowledge; however, philosophical assumptions are about insubstantial phenomena (beliefs and values) whereas scientific statements describe physical phenomena (1996, p. 56).

In 1979 the Representative Assembly passed Resolution C authorizing an extensive study. The Philosophical Base of Occupational Therapy Resolution stated:

The uniqueness of a profession is expressed in its philosophical base. Whereas, a philosophical base promotes a common professional identity; Whereas, the theoretical claims and practice methodologies of a profession are derived from a philosophical base; Whereas, a profession systematically engages in research in order to test those theories and methodologies. (*Occupational Therapy Newspaper*, January 1979, p. 5).

In the first project phase, academic program directors, faculty, and students identified seven philosophical themes (man, adaptation, role of education, quality of life, activity, contribution to society, and role function), when they reviewed occupational therapy literature from 1920 until 1978. Subsequent phases included further theme analysis according to historical timeframes. For example the dominant 1950s theme was man's relationship to his environment and work. The theme for the late 60 s and early 70 s was that man must have individual and societal involvement for satisfaction and worth. In project stage 4, Slagle lecturers reviewed and discussed these themes. The project ended in 1983 when Project Director Shannon submitted a January report to AOTA President Baum and AOTA's Executive Board and Representative Assembly for final approval. Writing about this work, Shannon stated the paper did not represent an official AOTA position, rather its purpose was "to trace the philosophical beliefs of the profession historically and to interpret those beliefs within the context of more modern times" (1993, p. 41). I think that Shannon interpreted the context of modern times through Reilly's occupational behavioral framework. As a Reilly protégé, Shannon used concepts like role behavior in the report and the following occupational behavior and/or Reilly-supported recommendations, stating:

> A shift in the profession's knowledge base from psychology and sociology to biology, social anthropology and social psychology (Shannon, 1983, p. 5927).
>
> Acute care is incompatible with occupational therapy's philosophy (Shannon, 1983, p. 5929).
>
> Multiple approaches to validating practice need to be explored within the context of a holistic philosophy (Shannon, 1983, p. 5932).

Eleven Eleanor Clarke Slagle lecturers deliberated occupational therapy's philosophical beliefs and knowledge development as it was thematically and historically grouped. Those attending "the Slagle meeting,"[53] in Arizona from July 12–16, 1982, were, in alphabetical order: Carolyn Baum (1980), Robert Bing (1981), Gail Fidler (1965), Alice Jantzen (1973), Jerry Johnson (1972), Lorna Jean King (1978), Mary Reilly (1961), Wilma West (1967), Ruth Weimer (1957), Elizabeth Yerxa (1966), and Muriel Zimmerman (1960). Carolyn Thomas, Philosophy Chair, The State University of New York consulted.[54] Occupational therapists Phillip Shannon and Denise Rotert were project director and assistant project director respectively. The "Slagle meeting" record contains professional lore and controversy. AOTA has sealed the meeting audiotapes, thus closing off potentially important information about occupational therapy's philosophical and theoretical foundations. Historically intriguing, what would drive a profession to seal its own records of the deliberations of such a highly respected group of scholars? In a February 7, 1983, letter from AOTA President Carolyn Baum to Project Director Phillip Shannon, and copied to AOTA Executive Director Jim Garibaldi and incoming AOTA President Bob Bing, Baum alluded to the tape sealing, stating: "I thank you for your support of the board's wishes regarding the 'tape issue' (Bing, private papers, 1983)."

What remains as public record from the project is Shannon's "Report on the AOTA Project to Identify the Philosophical Base of Occupational Therapy, condensed to "Toward a Philosophy of Occupational Therapy, August 1983." What remains privately however are personal minutes that Bing took during the meeting, providing a more comprehensive picture to a student of history. Bing, as AOTA president, became responsible for facilitating the record sealing. He gave the following full account, recalling:

> The archives that are locked away is [sic] not a pretty story. In 1983 we were still working on the philosophical base of OT. This project had been around for about 10 years, and not much had been completed. Mae Hightower–Vandamm, the president, wanted it finished before she left office: no such luck.[55] Carolyn [Baum] inherited it during her one year as president [1982–1983]. During the summer someone had the bright idea of gathering together a select group of former Eleanor Clarke Slagle lecturers and have them go over the report, and debate various issues that had been addressed in the philosophy. There were about 11 of us "invited" to this shindig in Phoenix in the middle of July. Hotter than the hinges of Hades. Mary Reilly, Gail Fidler, Wilma West, Betty Yerxa, Ruth Wiemer, Carolyn, me and 4 others met. I wrote a friend that first night that I felt I was the spear-carrier in some off-key grand opera and that I had wandered into the wrong theater. I really felt completely out of place.
>
> The very first thing was Mary Reilly loudly objecting to being taped. She did not want to be recorded. No real reason, just quirky. Everyone jumped all over her but she would not budge. We debated this for the first half of the day and came to a silly resolution. We could tape, however, there would be no transcript of the proceedings that would ever see the light of day. We agreed to this in order to get on with the job. I noticed that all of us were taking copious notes, more for protection than anything else.
>
> Then I became president and was handed this hot potato. I sought legal counsel from the AOTA lawyer and he said we could paraphrase what was said, but since we had agreed to Reilly's demands that the transcript be sealed, we had to go along with that. So we handed the project over to someone who had not been connected who did a summary, which got approved and passed on to the Representative Assembly. So far as I know the original transcripts, plus the tapes, are in a vault someplace. From time to time we do some really dumb things. (Bing/Peters oral history, February 23, 2003, lines 725–755)

The project's director, former Lieutenant Colonel Phillip D. Shannon, MA, MPA, Chief of occupational therapy, Academy of Health Sciences, Fort Sam Houston, Texas, in 1977, and chairman and associate professor of the Department of Occupational Therapy at the State University of New York,

Buffalo in 1983, had interesting community connections. Shannon was Reilly's former master's degree student at the University of Southern California (USC). Cromwell reported his Reilly mentorship, recalling:

> The military paid for the master's study for their people. Mary Reilly opened that route. We had a lot of military that came and got their master's with us at USC. Mary was hopeful about Phil (Shannon). He even got into a doctoral program but didn't finish. (Cromwell/Peters oral history, April 28–29, 2003, lines 3,046–3,049; 5,814–5,816)

Coordinating this AOTA project and other committee work, including an unsuccessful attempt at the AOTA presidency, Shannon was connected to other community members like Bing.[56] Bing, anticipating the Slagle meeting, wrote Shannon the following lighthearted letter:

> It should be a fascinating experience with all those prima donnas in one place and one time. I do hope you are planning on recording some or all of the proceeding; talk about archival material!
>
> Back in the mid- to late-60's the Association had a grant to prepare psychiatric OT's to teach, and Gail [Fidler] was the head of the project. We converged on New York State Psychiatric Institute for 2 weeks.[57] Mary Reilly showed up, I don't know if she was invited or if she just appeared. The result was absolutely fabulous, the dialogue, the confrontation. The sad part was that no one recorded all that. Maybe it was more like a Wagnerian opera with two prima donnas on stage at one time. I can hardly wait for the Phoenix "road show."
>
> I want to pick your brain about things that need changing, the invisibility of the male and how to correct that. We should have a good time together, protecting one another. (Letter to Shannon from Bing, June 24, 1982, Bing, private papers)

This letter highlighted Bing's outsider community status, identifying insiders as operatic stars and prima donnas and the gender barriers he felt as a male occupational therapist. Considering that Bing anticipated a Fidler and Reilly interchange, it is interesting that Fidler most remembered Reilly's attendance at the Slagle meeting. She recalled:

> Yes, I was part of that meeting. That was 'such' a show; we were all taken to a Scottsdale, Arizona hotel in July; it was hot as hell; the heat was unbearable. Phil (Shannon) organized it. They invited all the Eleanor Clarke Slagle lecturers, and they could have dispensed with most of them sitting around this table presenting an underlying philosophy of occupational therapy. I thought, good Lord, is this the way we do research? At which point Mary Reilly said, well there's one thing you need to have clear, I'm tired of being misquoted all the time, and I don't intend to open my mouth, I won't speak. I turned to Mary and said, "Why the hell did you

come; why are you here?" We limped and labored around and nobody had anything of substance to say. And that got sealed, that should have been wiped out and never existed. The content was zilch. Of course I can pontificate about what I thought the philosophy was, but that was mine. (Fidler/Peters oral history, March 6–7, 2003, lines 5,317–5,409)

Reviewing Bing's meeting notes, one sees that Reilly spoke more than others at the meeting. For example Bing noted Reilly speaking six times compared to Fidler's three or Johnson and Baum's two times out of a total of 17 comments.

Wiemer remembered not contributing due to the Arizona heat. Her Slagle meeting photographs showed how the community mixed work and social time, consistent with occupational therapy's insider culture. Those sitting poolside in the pictures included Mary Reilly; Harriett (Harry) Zlatohlavek, Reilly's housemate; Carolyn Baum; Lucie Murphy, an editor of the *American Journal of Occupational Therapy*; Willie (Wilma) West; Fred Sammons; Betty Yerxa; Ann Grady; and Gail (Fidler).[58] Weimer explained:

Scottsdale, that was a fascinating meeting, but I simply was nonfunctional at the time. When we flew in the night before, it must have been midnight, the pilot said it is now 102 degrees on the ground. Yes, I remember that I was so embarrassed that I was lost, and that I couldn't function because of the heat. Mary (Reilly) felt strongly about being taped.

That's why it was sealed. She felt it was nobody's business (about) what we were discussing. That perhaps the outcome could be formalized somehow, but the dialogue should not be. (Weimer/Peters oral history, March 18–19, 2003, lines 3,621–3,639; 3,607–3,616; 3,641–3,667)

Llorens, although invited, was unable to attend the meeting. Similar to Bing's feelings about regretting the sealing outcome, Llorens said:

The meeting is probably thematic to the contentiousness that does arise when we start to have a dialogue. I can tell you that part of the reason that it is sealed is some of the discussions that came about around Mary Reilly. I was not at the meeting, but yes, I think that is unfortunately the way in which too much has occurred. (Llorens/Peters oral history, April 25–26, 2003, lines 6,706–6,721)

Llorens further commented: "A lot of the philosophical base from the '70s that Shannon worked on came out of the Slagle meeting in Arizona (Llorens/Peters oral history, April 25–26, 2003, line 6,697–6,699)." Specifically, Shannon (1977) wrote about an occupational therapy's knowledge base "derailment."[59]

Fitting a philosophical framework, according to the agenda, addressed both the metaphysical (the nature of man) and epistemological position (how do we know?). Piecing together Bing's meeting notes, the agenda, and final report, one can reconstruct the meeting discussion.

Meeting discussion topics included research, professional trends like licensing, occupational therapy education, and treatment outcomes. Speaking about research and scientific replication, participants asked what is realistic in the traditional way of doing occupational therapy? Yerxa asked: how far should we go in adapting our research to a scientific model? Baum identified reductionistic research as a micro-view compared to macro-level multidisciplinary research.[60] Talking about making occupational therapy research available to a larger audience, Johnson stated, "It's not the uniqueness, but how the product is better than anyone else's. Fidler saw the issue being whether occupational therapists do it better than anyone else".

Looking toward occupational therapy education there was concern about where research fit into an overcrowded curriculum. Reilly saw this problem as systemic: "We have so much going on it's like putting on a neighborhood party while we are also putting out the fire which is consuming our house." Fidler, discussing a lack of autonomy from medicine said, "We're unwilling to take over our curricula, we keep tucking more in. Our tendency is to pick up something faddish and trendy; therapists don't question, they don't ask why." Reilly criticized occupational therapy's compliance saying, "anything anyone wants us to do, we do." (Bing, 1982). The final report summarized education discussions, suggesting three tiers. Entry-level education transmits knowledge and skills from the past. Master's level education has as it's purpose to study what has been and the doctoral level is to generate new knowledge (Shannon, 1983). Completing this 6.5-year segment in occupational therapy, the philosophical-based project wove philosophical assumptions like altruism with a need for scientific development. There were few lines drawn between occupational therapy science and philosophy.

AOTF: Funding Research and Science

Occupational therapy's research growth was connected to AOTF's founding on April 14, 1965, and the community of therapists who contributed their scholarship, efforts, and more concretely, found financial support. Where the association funded the Philosophical Base Project, the new foundation funded scientific research. The foundation furthered occupational therapy knowledge, theory, research, and scientific development. A milestone in occupational therapy's history, influential community members like West and Llorens directed the foundation's growth.

AOTF's 1967 President Yerxa (1967b) described the foundation's beginnings, asking the membership "how many times have you heard we need to do more research in OT?" (p. 299). Yerxa continued by identifying the profession's lack of money supporting such endeavors. Explaining AOTA's reorganization in 1964, spearheaded by AOTA President West, AOTF was established to "provide financial support to encourage scientific endeavor." (Yerxa, 1967b, p. 299). The foundation's board of directors outlined the following objectives for the Articles of Incorporation on October 1966:

> To advance the science of occupational therapy and increase the public knowledge and understanding thereof by the encouragement of the study of occupational therapy (1) through the provision of scholarships and fellowships ... (2) by engaging in studies, surveys and research, specifically to finance and conduct research studies to contribute to the body of knowledge of occupational therapy; and (3) by all other proper means; specifically to provide financial support .... (Yerxa, 1967b, p. 299)

Starting in November 1965, the association contributed $3,000 for legal and organizational funds and $177 came from association membership expenses. AOTF (1975), releasing a 10-year financial report summary, presented a fiscal summary that showed the growing organization as such:

Fund balance 6/30/66 ... $2,068.38
Fund balance 6/30/67 ... $38,275.84
Fund balance 6/30/70 ... $64,202.31
Fund balance 6/30/75 ... $155,488.00

On January 24, 1967, AOTF became a charitable and educational tax-exempt foundation (Internal Revenue Code 501C) which explains some of the growth between 1966 and 1967 financial figures (AOTF, 1975; Yerxa, 1967b). In 1967 AOTA transferred approximately $13,335 in bequests and memorial funds to AOTF. Secondly, in 1967, the Delegate Assembly approved allocating a yearly sum in the AOTA budget for the foundation's operating expenses. It wasn't however until June 1969 that 2% of AOTA's annual dues was allocated (AOTF, 1975).

As a resourceful person during the 1960s, AOTA Executive Director Marjorie Fish between 1952 until 1965, working with fellow Boston School graduate and AOTA President West from 1961 until 1964, found government funding through the Departments of Health and Vocational Rehabilitation. Llorens remembered participating in various workshops in the 1960s. She stated:

> I was invited by Wilma West to some workshops and with Fidler, the Walden Woods, Michigan workshops about object relations. I think it was the combined sponsorship of Wilma West and Marge Fish; it was Rehab sponsored, SRA (Social Rehabilitation Administration) between 1965 and 1967. We were looking at the theoretical and conceptual aspects of activities and objects. We had to bring an object that had a lot of meaning, and talk about it. It also involved projective techniques, Azima's work. The third one in the trilogy was the Albion, Michigan

workshop. That one involved Fidler, Mosey, and Kovalenko, and others. That was an effort at trying to bring about dialogue about the issues of activit[ies] and their importance. (Llorens/Peters oral history, April 25–26, 2003, lines 6,555–6,629)

In the 1970s the foundation grew, as did research development monies. In 1975 an AOTA–AOTF research development program to assist in developing objectives and defining research projects for occupational therapy researchers was funded for $10,000 (AOTF, 1975). West funneled these funds into continuing education workshops. One example was a pediatric sensory/perceptual motor themed workshop in 1978. Gilfoyle and Llorens remembered the workshop because it involved 20 therapists. Gilfoyle said:

We weren't trained in research; none of us really wanted to go back to school and give up our practices. It was too exciting. We had a one-week course, and Willie (West) helped us find and invite 20 therapists. Jean Ayres was there to teach research, Jo Moore was there and Ken Hopkins, a statistician from the University of Colorado. Facilitator mentors were matched to the 20 therapists. Anne Henderson was a mentor. The therapists presented their projects in San Francisco one year later, giving a 10-minute synopsis of their research. It was the first research symposium we ever had. Looking back, that was part of my legacy; that was the true beginnings in getting clinicians involved in research. It was because of Willie, and what Jean Ayres had done. It was about empowering people, that people can do it, you don't have to have a PhD, we can just do it. (Gilfoyle/Peters oral history, February 10–11, 2003, lines 874–918)

Llorens remembered:

We did try to do some research that was like a community. It was fueled by the development of the research grant program in the foundation. It was a fledgling effort at creating a research program. Each of us had four or five people to mentor through the process. We had 20 therapists engaged in research all around the country. They took a year to do their study. These were practitioners; Linda Faria had an excellent paper: 'The developmental observations of offsprings of parents ingesting illicit LSD.' Elizabeth Danella was one of my graduate students in Florida, Mary Kawar, and Wanda Mayberry were others. I believe that was probably the first concerted effort that I can remember, that I was involved in, of occupational therapists making an effort to start to do research that was theory based, to try to establish some science. (Llorens/Peters oral history, April 25–26, 2003, lines 2,887–2,936; 2,624–2,635)

Newly funded, the community of therapists participated in and/or taught various workshops and seminars about research. Nedra Gillette, AOTF's director of research for approximately 30 years, remembered the mid-1970s foundation workshops, saying "At first we did workshops around the country. Betty Yerxa volunteered right off the bat, 'Research begins with a small r.' It was an effort not to terrify people." (Gillette/Peters interview, January 29, 2003, lines 1,303–1,307).

Llorens remembered another West invitation-based workshop that Fidler facilitated in the 1970s, recalling:

> There was some dialogue amongst theorists at "Exploring How a Think Feels." Gail Fidler was involved in that and Mosey. That was related to another Wilma West invitation. She brought us all together to talk about mental health. What we were essentially trying to do was think about theories of activity performance. We tried to articulate the emotional and physical underpinnings of occupational therapy. (Llorens/Peters oral history, April 25–26, 2003, lines 6,369–6,383; 2,701–2,713)

Expanding scholarship funding, the foundation sponsored grant writing workshops, the first in 1975 at AOTA's annual conference in Milwaukee (AOTF, 1975). Gillette spoke about formalizing research efforts through the foundation's Research Advisory Council. She stated:

> Lela (Llorens) chaired the Research Advisory Council the first 10 years of its life. That was a structure that she and Ann Grady, Willie (West), and I built. The council included the chair and chairs of four committees. They were the grants review, publications that led to starting the *Occupational Therapy Journal of Research*, and the think tank, which was the Research Development Committee. (Gillette/Peters interview, January 29, 2003, lines 1,590–1,608)

Remembering her work with the Research Advisory Council, Llorens talked about the think tank atmosphere that Gillette referred to, saying:

> We talked about a dual mission of research in practice contributing to the development of a body of knowledge and helping to sustain clinical practice. That was our mission. I think the foundation's mission was pretty clear. The research part was to educate the profession to the needs for research and to disseminate that research for use by practitioners. Our goal was to legitimize a profession through research, publications, and contributions to the world.
> We would schedule meetings to do brainstorming, plan to prepare for workshops or seminars, because that was a new direction. (Llorens/Peters oral history, April 25–26, 2003, lines 4,715–4772; 4,608–4,634)

This section addressed AOTF and AOTA leaders roles in funding research. The community of therapists combined their efforts to help develop occupational therapy's unique body of knowledge. People like West and Fish found funding sources; Llorens, Yerxa, and colleagues formed occupational therapy's think tank; and leaders Fidler and Gilfoyle spearheaded innovative occupational therapy practice that was supported by government grants.

This section reviewed how the community of therapists defined occupational therapy knowledge as philosophically- or scientifically-based, which are divergent viewpoints, and thus created a dilemma that continues to influence the profession today. Therapists supporting a philosophic viewpoint, like humanism, identified with feminine caring, serving, and nurturing (Morantz–Sanchez, 1985, 1997). Therapists supporting science, like the medical model, aligned with an objective male viewpoint.[61] As occupational therapy developed from the 1950s, philosophy and science created subtle differences in occupational therapy's treatment emphasis, knowledge development, and professional direction.

Occupational therapy's philosophical foundation was rooted to the meaning and purpose of therapeutic activities to the individual. These core values combined with occupational therapy leaders' beliefs that productive activity or occupation facilitated a productive life remain a valued aspect of occupational therapy's identity and work. For example, Stattel said:

> I think we have been a mixture of always questioning who we are. I don't think that is bad. We must retain what we felt; we were humanitarians, we were concerned with the whole person. We must get the body, mind, and spirit or if you will, soul together. (Stattel/Peters oral history, November 20, 1997, lines 640–645)

Insider occupational therapy leaders in the community of therapists prioritized occupational therapy's philosophical base, with AOTA funding a 6.5 project (six years, six months) in the 1970s that is discussed later in this section. Interestingly, there were no parallel studies about the importance of occupational therapy's scientific knowledge base from 1950 until 1980.

More curiously today, in an age of science and efficacy, occupational therapy's leadership continues to invest time and resources toward studying occupational therapy's philosophical foundation. For example, in an AOTA draft report from Mary M. Evert, a former AOTA president serving in the capacity as the speaker to the Representative Assembly (RA); and Kathlyn L. Reed,[62] Ad Hoc Foundation's Committee Chairperson; and Texas representative to the AOTA RA dated May 4, 2004, a motion was adopted in the RA in 2003 to study the historical foundations of the profession. The RA has supported the "foundations" study through 2006, which has brought together 1986 Slagle lecturer Reed, and 2005 Slagle lecturer Suzanne Peloquin during the first year of the project (Reed to Ad Hoc Foundations Committee Member Peters correspondence, Peters private collection, 2004).

Discussions about science in occupational therapy were limited and community outsider dominated, with some insiders agreeing, emerging in the 1960s and 1970s (Mosey, 1981; Reilly, 1960; Yerxa, 1974). This was parallel to Kuhn's (1970) view supporting a new interpretation of traditional science, and paradigm shifts. Community scholars like Ayres, Llorens, Mosey, and Reilly began questioning and challenging sciences' relationship to occupational therapy practice. They developed occupational therapy theories and guidelines for practice that provided a much-needed foundation that better-informed occupational practice, and helped therapists articulate how they served society. Seeking rationales about why what they did worked, some members in the community asked and sought new answers. For example Bing described his perspective about scientific justification while teaching at the University of Florida in 196, stating:

> The main thing I tried to get across was the 'why' of what we did and less the 'what.' I felt that an OT had to always explain to the patient or the M.D. why we were doing some of the things we did, that would appear silly or child-like to others. (Bing/Peters oral history, February 26, 2003, lines 917–921)

Yerxa, supporting a scientific knowledge base view in the 1960s and 1970s added:

> I define a science-based profession differently today than I would have in the 60s or 70s. I thought that traditional science was going to validate what we did. I would enable us to publicize by writing about it, and in a sense prove our efficacy. But I don't think that occupational therapy lends itself to that kind of science at all. Any science that supports occupational therapy has to take into account the person's consciousness, the culture, and social system. (Yerxa/Peters oral history, April 21–22, 2003, lines 3,694–3,769; 2,152–2,186)

Yerxa's changing views paralleled changes that occurred in occupational therapy knowledge development. I agree with her reflection that the nature of occupational therapy knowledge shifted, and further propose in the next section that these changes occurred because of specific social and historical events.

Old-guard sustainers and political community insiders like Stattel and Wiemer, supporting a philosophically-based occupational therapy knowledge view, strongly believed a humanistic doctrine represented occupational therapy's core, similar to a global or uniform theory. They thought that every person, regardless of disability, or life challenges could live a productive and purposeful life. Occupational therapy outsider theorists like Ayres, Mosey, and Rood also believed in these values, but questioned whether a belief system was all that occupational therapy needed to evolve to a scholarly discipline. Creating a unique body of knowledge, they contributed a theoretical and scientific approach to treatment that ultimately shifted the profession's direction.

Challenging the occupational therapy philosophical viewpoint, those supporting a more scientific approach to practice professed that occupational therapy could better serve society by developing a deeper understanding of not only the why, or altruistic caring, but the theoretical how of what the profession did. Thus, a dilemma emerged, particularly in the 1960s and 1970s. This coincided with occupational therapy's 1970s exploration into specialization. Specialization, modeled after medicine and science, was occupational therapy's attempt to divide and expand expert knowledge into specific clinical areas like neurology, pediatrics, and psychiatry. Although specialty and a scientific approach to practice is present today in occupational therapy, a philosophical approach to practice remains extremely important. Occupational therapy leaders and Slagle lecturers presently discuss core values, and the meaning of occupation or activity. Therefore, the occupational therapy science and philosophy pendulum continues to shift with little consensus or resolution about professional direction amongst leaders.

Secondly, implied in the division between philosophy and science is an inherent division between the characteristically feminine caring and masculine science in a predominantly female profession. Establishing a tension in the community, the outsider theorists and futurists, braving a less popular viewpoint, supported science, and braving these untreaded waters, may have added to their exclusionary status.

Those therapists criticizing an objective or cold scientific approach, were concerned that it did not factor in the importance of caring. A point worthy of discussion, but debate was not part of occupational therapy's community culture. More disconcerting, leaders were cutting off or excluding important internal dialogue, arguments, and critisms needed to academically mature the profession. The philosophy/science dilemma established a precedent for similar questions today about professional development and the place for founding values in an efficacy driven health care system. For example, one question worth discussing is whether it is the heart or head of practice that today's therapist seek? Llorens opened the window to this debate in the following analysis where she explained how science differed from the meaning or art of practice, stating:

> Practice has a meaning component to the individual receiving therapy and engaging in therapy. Whereas science has more detachment, you have to maintain a certain amount of objectivity to account for what you are seeing in a way that is credible. We have a lot more experience with practice than research. (Llorens/Peters oral history, April 25–26, 2003, lines 4,436–4,446)

Spearheaded by West and Llorens, the foundation shifted the philosophy verses science pendulum from philosophy to a midpoint or balance that presently leans towards science (Gilfoyle & Christiansen, 1987; Llorens, 1981a; West, 1981). West, a community insider, believed that developing knowledge was a way to legitimize the profession (Cox & West, 1982). Occupational therapy's knowledge development, however, was thwarted because community insiders and outsiders held different visions for occupational therapy's direction.

Community insiders maintained that occupational therapy's knowledge should be philosophically based, that reflected the founding principles of caring. Community outsiders believed that science would better expand the profession, and would provide the needed theoretical foundation for practice to better serve patients. Insiders opposed this view, saying science was too cold and objective, and did not reflect occupational therapy's humanistic core. An internal dilemma developed, and was identified as a system disturbance in the system of professions. Although dialogue and debate may have aided a consensus, it was not part of the community culture. Professional growth was thwarted, and resources were divided between those supporting a philosophical foundation, and those supporting a scientific basis for practice. Secondly, although occupational therapy leaders like West, Fidler, Gilfoyle, and Yerxa believed that a theoretical foundation for practice was important, they questioned whether the larger membership utilized and understood the importance of theory to practice.

Theory development expanded occupational therapists' ability to better understand that practice was not isolated, but rather was supported by theory and research, and that patients would reap the benefits. I believe the larger membership integrated theory into their practice by the 1980s, but it required a continual leadership effort and consensus over 30 years to happen. Such efforts included identifying a cadre of scholars, theory and research development; continuing education workshops; and funding scholarly efforts. These efforts remained in the political hands of a few like Wilma West, Marjorie Fish, and other community insiders. Insiders knew, however, that they needed occupational therapy scholars, who were the community outsiders, to develop and expand occupational therapy's expert knowledge. Objectively, occupational therapy's landscape changed, and occupational therapy owned its own knowledge base by 1980, but a change to science was not readily embraced. The next section summarizes occupational therapy in the larger system of professions and the external social movements.

SECTION VII: PROFESSIONALIZING: OCCUPATIONAL THERAPY AND SOCIAL MOVEMENTS

Occupational therapists, characterized in the 1950s as health care workers who entertained patients, shucked their dated crafts ladies image and expanded their influence beyond occupational therapy clinics located in hospital basements. Striving for independence and professionalism, leaders shunned medicine's characteristically paternalistic 40-year dominance in the late 1960s and 1970s. How did a small community of therapists, mostly women, covertly fight for the independence which changed the face of occupational therapy at a time when women stayed in the shadows of male professionals? Goal-directed to uniquely help patients, therapists strategized their position in the larger system of profession and society. Doing as they saw fit, at the core, occupational therapy scholars and leaders were powerful women (Cromwell, line 5664; Yerxa, lines 1866, 3204), who used their talents shrewdly (Cromwell, 1959, 1977, 1985). Establishing priorities, political power took precedence over knowledge development, so that occupational therapy was viable enough to survive competition from other health care professions.

This section explores how the community of therapists capitalized upon American social reform movements, including the rehabilitation and equal rights movements, to expand the profession. Building partnerships with other health care professionals, the community of therapists gained autonomy and enhanced occupational therapy's viability.

The conservative larger membership did not rally for dramatic change, or completely sever medicine's (male) domination. Leaders knew that breaking away from medicine's traditional ties required behind the scenes maneuvers. The most political leaders like Wiemer, Cromwell, and Fidler, knew what they had to do to challenge competitors successfully. Who were occupational therapy's competitors? Certainly not the more established health care professionals like physicians, psychologists, nurses, or social workers. Rather, occupational therapy leaders partnered and struggled with other allied health professionals like physical therapists; speech pathologists; corrective therapists; art, music, and dance therapists; and recreation therapists. For example, I uncovered in a folder entitled "Erosion," that included letters written to leaders of other health disciplines, like the American Medical Association and American Nurses' Association (ANA), between 1978 until 1981, by AOTA President Mae Hightower–Van Damn, AOTA Executive Director Jim Garabaldi, and 1978 chairman of the Coalition of Independent Health Professions (CIHP). The correspondence addressed turf war battles between occupational therapy and art therapy, corrective therapy, and physical therapy. Garabaldi received support from ANA Director of Practice Roma Lee Taunton, in a December 20, 1978 letter, that discussed a concern about prevention of fragmentation of patient care (Crampton private papers, 1978). More pointedly, Hightower–Van Damn received a letter from a frustrated occupational therapist and Clinical Department Chief Marilyn C. Ryan, of the Ohio Department of Mental Health and Mental Retardation that stated her feelings about occupational therapy's infringements, stating:

> Teachers and psychologists feel that ADL [activities of daily living] is their turf and invention, and that Marc Gold is the inventor of task analysis and rehabilitation counselors' pre-vocational evaluation. I feel that there is little that is unique to OT [occupational therapy] anymore, except that

OT can have a broader spectrum of knowledge that others lack. OTs are not an aggressive breed like many PTs [physical therapists]. Would it not be good to have someone looking at the marketing aspect? Some of that grinds my soul as a professional. What happened to the concept of the discipline having expert knowledge? (Letter from Ryan to Hightower–Vandamn, May 20, 1980; Cramton private papers, 1980)

Concerned about erosion or turf infringement, leaders befriended legislators, administrators, other health care professionals, and academics, to educate them about occupational therapy's merits. For example Cromwell remembered building political alliances in the now disbanded CIHP. Cromwell, the second coalition chairperson in 1974 talked about her CIHP involvement from 1969 until 1974, recalling:

The coalition was the attempt in Washington to get the health disciplines to put their heads together. We came together to have a combined voice to influence legislation and try to impact health. Everybody but medicine was there: nursing, psychology, social work, PT [physical therapy], OT [occupational therapy], dietitians, osteopaths, optometrists, podiatrists and lab technicians. Ruth Wiemer was the first one on the board. It was about Medicare legislation, grants and the fringes, the podiatrists and osteopaths. We were trying to figure out how we could have an impact. (Cromwell/Peters oral history, April 28–29, 2003, lines 6,601–6,606; 6,385–6,475)

These political maneuvers took precedence over expanding professional knowledge. As stated earlier, knowledge was not all that was needed to make occupational therapy known in a larger social and political context. Therapists had to first gain autonomy and power to own their profession.

Using a network, they scouted new opportunities and trends in health care and public policy, and connected to the "right" people in influential positions in government, academia, and health care. Like their occupational therapy teachers, these predominantly middle and upper-middle class white women had the "can do" spirit. Stattel captured this essence when she stated:

The war [World War II] brought out the importance of women in the running of local society. It was the Second World War that brought forth women like Ruth Robinson. She was just a marvelous president of AOTA. There was Carlotta Welles who knew Signe Brunstrumm. All of those women got together and were dealing at a different (higher) level. (Stattel/Peters oral history, November 20, 1997, lines 681–686)

A unique knowledge base legitimized occupational therapy as a profession, but community leaders held the key that opened the political doors to gain their autonomy.

Social Movements and Occupational Therapy

Occupational therapy gained health care jurisdiction or clout through a chain of events, or interactions that occurred when community members combined their interests in social movements, like the women's movement and the work to make occupational therapy a bona fide profession with a unique body of knowledge (Figure 4). Summarizing occupational therapy changes that occurred over 30 years, community power shifts went from the conservative old-guard sustainers and political movers who appreciated physician's mentoring in the 1950s, to a strong statement of autonomy by 1980. Outsider theorists and new-guard sustainers, along with more radical political movers and futurists made their professional mark in the 1970s. Forward thinkers and identified feminists sought a theoretically-based foundation to practice to better serve patients, and in so doing, created a newfound professional identity.

The 1950s rehabilitation movement, depicted in Figure 4, was a social movement that suggested that reconditioning, retraining, and purposeful work should be available to individuals suffering from physical and mental disabilities, and in turn, create opportunities for occupational therapists. Community insiders, military leaders, and old-guard sustainers politely

Social Movements and Occupational Therapy's Professionalization

Social Movement	Knowledge	Relationships	Community Involvement
1950s Rehabilitation	Pragmatic Trial and error Problem solving	Physicians dominate and mentor occupational therapists' knowledge development Hospital-based	Military leaders influence AOTA Old guard insiders and sustainers
1960s Equal Rights Disability	External theories guide occupational therapy intervention	Works with other therapies (physical, creative arts, and recreational therapies Community-based treatment	Political Insiders make strides Insiders and futurists voice opinions
1970s Women's Movement /Feminism	Unique occupational therapy theories and frames of reference	Autonomy, independent and internally diverse	Outsider theorists and futurists seek new direction

FIGURE 4 Occupational therapy gains jurisdiction through a chain of events.

charged the gates, making occupational therapy's worth known to legislators, administrators, and physicians involved in the rehabilitation movement, thus starting a chain of events.

Physicians appointed themselves occupational therapy mentors and teachers in the 1950s and 1960s. Dominating occupational therapy's knowledge development, physician's proposed a scientific foundation. Complying, occupational therapists, taught to respect and defer to physician's authority and status in occupational therapy school, developed knowledge and treatment that was pragmatic, and used a trial-and-error approach to solve patient's problems.

Occupational therapists, shifting their views, gained a new voice in the social reforms-oriented 1960s, where ideally, people with disabilities, people of color, and women earned equal respect, opportunities, and pay. Community insiders, particularly the political movers, educated others about occupational therapy's role in helping the disenfranchised. Occupational therapy's futurists saw social reform as an excellent opportunity to broaden the profession's platforms. Joining with other health care professionals, like physical therapists, creative arts therapists, and recreation therapists, occupational therapy leaders began to engage in theoretical dialogues. Occupational therapists began articulating their expert knowledge with psychologists, educators, and physical therapists. Therapists discussed Freud, Kabot, and Gesell's theoretical work to support practice. Creating a bridge, using a common theoretical vocabulary with other disciplines, occupational therapists became integrated members of multi-disciplinary treatment teams.

Leaders ventured out, entering new work environments. Directly related to the 1960s disabilities movement and increased social awareness, therapists were no longer limited to hospital-based practice. Occupational therapists worked at newly developed centers for independent living and community mental health programs. This increased occupational therapy's visibility, and expanded the need for services. The 1960s occupational therapy transitions continued into the 1970s, when therapists entered the public school system in numbers. Parent's began understanding that occupational therapy helped their children's school performance, and became newfound advocates at school board meetings, and when talking to their elected officials about services.

The women's movement in the 1970s changed women's opportunities. Community members Fidler, Gilfoyle, Johnson, and Yerxa strongly believed the women's movement positively influenced the profession (Johnson, 1978). Debatable amongst the most conservative who deny involvement, like Crampton and Welles, middle class white women, following Friedan's (1963) lead, joined efforts to counter women's dependent stereotypes. Ironically, independent competent professionals Crampton, and Welles, did not identify with feminist doctrine, but represented in their actions the essence of the movement.

Savvy leaders and scholars had an eye toward change. Change meant that people of color and male occupational therapists, less than a handful, started to gain community entrance. Change also meant that outsider theorists set the profession's intellectual agenda, supporting a move toward a science rather than a philosophically-based profession. Occupational therapy moving forward still had roadblocks to solve. For example, shifting away from medicine carried with it internal professional confusion and tension. Those supporting a philosophically based practice, the old guard insiders, didn't value a shift toward science. Traditional old guard community insiders supported medicine's umbrella, while a 1960s' liberal insider and outsider group platformed for independence.

Roadblocks also occurred between community leaders and the larger membership. For example, occupational therapy leaders made decisions that were not always understood or supported by the larger membership. The membership believed medicine was occupational therapy's good shepherd, and any split was unfounded. Colman (1984) studied divisions between eaders and the membership that she identified as an elite and proletariat class distinction in occupational therapy. She believed a small group of women, academic program directors, guided and controlled the profession's pulse. I agree with Colman's analysis, and expand it by stating that academic program directors, like Wade, Willard, Green, Fish, and Spear extended their influence beyond academe by forming a network of women. They were capable women who were in the right place at the right time, exploring opportunities from the 1960s women's movement. The community of therapists surpassed their mentors as departmental chairpersons, gaining academic vice president and provost appointments like Llorens and Gilfoyle. On another path, West, Wiemer, Crampton, and Fidler held federal and state health administrative jobs. Making their mark, these women determined AOTAs and AOTFs direction for 30 years.

Chain of Events: Rehabilitation and Equal Rights

Starting a chain of events (Abbott, 1988), community insiders positioned occupational therapy in the health care marketplace, with physicians, psychologists, social workers, nurses, physical therapists, speech pathologists, recreational and creative arts therapists, corrective therapists, vocational counselors, educators, patients, and legislatures. Attuned to national trends, scholars and leaders monitored occupational therapy's place in the rehabilitation and equal rights movements of the 1960s. For example, in 1975, marking the United Nation's theme "international year for women," and the foundation's 10th anniversary, the *American Journal of Occupational Therapy* devoted the November–December issue to women's issues. Articles addressed "being female and the ramifications on the choice of and practice of (occupational therapy) as a health profession" (Viseltear, 1975, p. 641).

Prior to the 1960s equal rights movement, the social and political rehabilitation movement acted as an external social force or agent in the system of professions.[63,64] Addressing constituency needs following World War II, Congress established the Department of Medicine and Surgery in the Veterans Administration (VA), and the VA's Vocational Rehabilitation and Education services (Dean, 1972). The VA's physical medicine and rehabilitation services, spearheaded by Dr. Howard Rusk, included occupational and physical therapy, speech pathology, manual arts therapy, and educational therapy, thus making occupational therapy a team member. Rusk's wartime medical experiences laid the foundation for his post-war years' work at the Institute of Rehabilitation and Physical Medicine (IRM) in New York, starting in 1948. In 1950, occupational therapist and 1960 Slagle recipient Muriel Zimmerman worked at IRM, starting her more than 25-year tenure. IRM became a rehabilitation research institution in 1962 as part of New York University. Zimmerman, joining fellow community members and Philadelphia School alumni Stattel and Behlen, taught courses at the New York University Department of Occupational Therapy from 1956 until 1974. Yerxa remembered Zimmerman's attending a course in 1957 or 1958 that Yerxa helped develop at Rancho Los Amigos National Rehabilitation Center.[65] Yerxa remembered Zimmerman's reputation in occupational therapy, stating:

> Muriel Zimmerman was famous in OT; she worked at Rusk and was the epitome of hand splinting knowledge. When we designed this course with UCLA, they invited people from all over the United States to take the course and evaluate what we were presenting. Muriel Zimmerman was invited as well as people from Warm Springs, which was the big epiphany in those days. Here I am this little pipsqueak, 27 or 28 years old and it was like God coming; she was so highly thought of. She was very kind and gentle, but we didn't know what she was going to be like. (Yerxa/Peters oral history, April 21–22, 2003, lines 1,517–1,549)

IRM was one of two early centers that linked clinical teaching to rehabilitation research, the other at the University of Minnesota (Dean, 1972; Gritzer & Arluke, 1985). Cromwell remembered Minnesota's 1960s rehabilitation medicine reputation, saying: "Minnesota was a haven of physiatry; they controlled everything in physical medicine. We struggled, helping OT's survive who had physiatrist bosses (Cromwell/Peters oral history, April 28–29, 2003, lines 1,894–1,907)."

In the 1960s other rehabilitation research centers gained research clout and dollars, including Baylor University and the Texas Institute of Rehabilitation, Temple University in Pennsylvania, the University of Colorado, and the University of Southern California's affiliation with Rancho Los Amigos. Occupational therapists working at these centers, like Zimmerman and Yerxa, were active research team members. The Vocational Rehabilitation Act, 1964, applied federal dollars to support training grants in such areas as vocational evaluation and work adjustment (Gritzer & Arluke, 1985). By the late 1960s, occupational therapists West and Fidler, among others, tapped into these sources for AOTA, using the monies for workshop training and graduate education. Yerxa, according to her self-report, and Mosey, earned their doctorate degrees at Boston University and New York University respectively during the 1960s, based on these resources. Fidler spoke about capturing grant funds, recalling:

> I wrote a lot of grants, spent half the night sitting in my (AOTA) office until 3 or 4 o'clock in the morning. I wrote grants for PhDs and for the certification examination project. That was all rehabilitation. Rehab dried up, but those were great years, being able to sit down and spend a night writing a grant, and the next morning sending it in and saying I have $150,000 coming. I was the first one who did that other than Willie (West), who was in the system. I remember that it was $900,000 in federal grants that I had written in one year. (Fidler/Peters oral history, March 6–7, 2003, lines 2,097–2,114; 2,307–2,315)

It was fascinating for the time, that Fidler, who had a post-baccalaureate occupational therapy certificate, was able to garner these federal grants, customarily open to doctoral-level professionals in other disciplines. Was this more a commentary about Fidler, the woman, or her entrances to known physicians like her husband, or the developing status of the profession? My analysis is that it was a little about everything.

Expanding the rehabilitation movement, public health physicians and nurses led the "war on germs" and infectious disease in the early 1950s. Occupational therapists worked with tuberculosis and poliomyelitis patients who came from all socioeconomic and cultural backgrounds. Both poor and immigrant tenement housing residents, and America's middle class children, became ill with poliomyelitis, expanding to epidemic proportions in the 1950s until the Salk vaccine defeated the virus (Brandt, 1997; Brown, 1997; Starr, 1982; Tomes, 1998). Yerxa remembered working with poliomyelitis patients at Rancho Los Amigos National Rehabilitation Center in Los Angeles, saying:

> People who worked in polio always looked to Georgia, Warm Springs, but they had passed their peak and Rancho became the peak. I went to Rancho in 1956. I walked onto a ward in a long old barrack building, probably 75 feet long, and it was just tank respirators. We had people who could only move one muscle. Great advances happened so that people could get out of the tank respirators. (Yerxa/Peters oral history, April 21–22, 2003, lines 1,558–1,618; 1,356–1,419)

With health care needs taking priority, funding programs like those from the Department of Vocational Rehabilitation, and private funding from organizations like the National Foundation for Infantile Paralysis helped establish occupational therapy's rehabilitation role and an increasing demand for services (Kahmann, 1950). Bing explained the changes in occupational therapy's domain, stating:

> The benchmark of the 1950s was vocational rehabilitation. During World War II, and later, the VA had OT and PT under physical medicine. Two additional groups were created, corrective therapy and manual arts therapy. Military hospitals during the Korean War had these corrective therapists. Amendments to the Vocational Rehabilitation Act helped create rehab units as stand-alone institutions or as units within large hospitals. A whole new profession arose, vocational counselors, who struggled with pre-vocational evaluation using work samples. Monies became available for large-scale workshops to retrain OTs to fit into the new scheme of things.
>
> There was also an awakening to children's needs for our services in the 1950s. The child development movement in education spilled over so that chronically ill kids became part of our domain. Tuberculosis as a chronic, long-term disease was eradicated. We had to make considerable adjustments in our thinking and doing about chronicity. (Bing/Peters oral history, February 6, 2003, lines 50–79)

Bing's 1950s occupational therapy overview highlights a growth period. In the system of professions, however, this growth also meant increased marketplace competition amongst various rehabilitation therapists (occupational therapy, physical therapy, vocational counselors, and corrective therapists) jockeying for their existence and health care dollars.

Medicine, leading the pack in American health care claimed a new sense of optimism from 1950 until 1980 (Starr, 1982). Having clout, physicians sought new political and financial relationships, aligning with health insurance companies and labor unions to fund research and medical education (Starr, 1982). Exclusivity was one way that medicine claimed autonomy; science was the other road to authority.[66] As with occupational therapists gaining their place amongst other rehabilitation therapists, physicians learned that doctors of homeopathy, osteopathy, optometry, and chiropractic were speaking about testing alternative medicine hypotheses and extending knowledge (Gevitz, 1988). Seeking new research alliances, occupational therapist Ayres connected with optometrists. Cromwell remembered:

> Jean Ayres got interested in perceptual motor problems, and she worked with optometrists. They were more interested in the visual perceptual kinds of things than ophthalmologists ever were. The ophthalmologists didn't know what she was talking about; they weren't interested in the same kinds of things about children that Jean was interested in. She persisted and had a cadre of local optometrists in the San FernandoValley that she did research with. (Cromwell/Peters oral history, April 28–29, 2003, lines 1,911–1,925)

Medicine's counter to these alternative medicine infringements was to maintain a male-dominated scientific authority. Using this strategy, physicians produced empirical research supported by federal and private funding; thus they gained access to political and social reimbursement systems (Starr, 1982).[67]

Physicians, as project directors, awarded government-sponsored grants, and determined the multidisciplinary research team, including occupational therapists. In these environments, therapists like Gilfoyle furthered their expertise and met other community members participating in research. Gilfoyle remembered her early days at Craig Rehabilitation Center in Denver and the medical director who spurred her research interests, stating:

> I was at Craig late 1959, or early 1960, and that was during the thalido-mide government contract days. The medical director, John Young, he was a real mentor, sent me to Rancho Los Amigos and UCLA where I took post-graduate courses in prosthetics and orthotics. This was my first involvement with research. That's when I met Betty Yerxa, Lois Barber, and Dottie Wilson. I was there for almost two months and we became good friends. Royce Nelson was the orthotist in charge at Rancho. Lois Barber was the OT that [sic] was working with him doing research, and I was down in that lab all the time developing things. It was a great opportunity. (Gilfoyle/Peters oral history, February 10–11, 2003, lines 266–271; 401–430; 509–524)

Medical science, characterized as reductionistic in rationale (Yerxa, 1983), and objective in outlook was identified as male thinking (Ludmerer, 1999; Morantz–Sanchez, 1997, 1985). This had ramifications for the predominantly female occupational therapy. Separation from medicine meant that occupational therapists needed to be responsible for their autonomy. Yerxa and Fidler talked about the perceived dependency between male physicians and female occupational therapists as a father/daughter relationship. Yerxa stated:

> It was either medicine was going to tell us what we were going to do, or we were going to be autonomous. If we were going to be autonomous, then we'd better know what we were talking about. We had better have a strong base of knowledge in order to demonstrate our efficacy. It was a father/daughter kind of thing. (Yerxa/Peters oral history, April 21–22, 2003, lines 3,629–3,639)

Fidler added:

> We want to be doctors. I think that's why we take such pot shots at physicians, only to turn around and behave exactly the way we accused them of behaving. I was at fault too. I can remember when people would ask me what I do in a non-OT audience, I would say I'm a psychiatric

occupational therapist, OT was always very quiet under my breath. Psychiatry was my ticket to credibility. Psychologically, the doctor is daddy, it's one of those female things. (Fidler/Peters oral history, March 6–7, 2003, lines 6,149–6,700)

Yerxa and Fidler presented two ends of the spectrum, therapists wanting autonomy, yet, finding some credibility and security remaining under medicine's power. This push–pull process influenced occupational therapists professional identity.

Some occupational therapists in the community of therapists making inroads and career gains worked well alongside noted physicians entering mentorships and partnerships. Gilfoyle overcame the male doctor and female occupational therapist stereotype stating:

I gained respect from the male physicians for being who I was, and feeling their equal. That comes from my father, I think. I never felt like a victim, or like we were victims of the medical profession. (Gilfoyle/Peters oral history, February 10–11, 2003, lines 1,081–1,087)

Traditionally established, various community members entered positive working relationships with physicians. Wiemer explained:

Our early people were very comfortable with physicians. Look at the founders in Clifton Springs; Kidner, Barton, Johnson, and Dunton, and the first presidents, a lot of them men from 1917 through 1946. Other than Mrs. Slagle, there were physicians for years. It was a comfortable leadership. Interestingly, the females turned to the males for leadership in those days. (Wiemer/Peters oral history, March 18–19, 2003, lines 6,579–6,609)

Proving educational for all, therapist Bing grew close to physician Dunton; therapist Crampton worked with physician Solomon; therapist Fidler respected physicians Noyes and Fidler; Stattel worked with physician Kessler; therapist Brunyate Wiemer worked with physician Phelps and remained friends with Dunton; and Yerxa worked with Nickel. Stattel remembered how Kessler supported occupational therapy exposure in the mid-1950s in New Jersey, saying:

At Kessler we had a PR [public relations] person who was promoting me like mad. I couldn't stop her, I didn't want to. Dr. Kessler wanted all that; everywhere I went I had publicity. (Stattel/Peters oral history, November 20, 1997, lines 6,671–6,674)

Wiemer remembered the career opportunities she experienced because of alliances with physicians. These experiences included publishing with

Dunton, her years with Phelps, and her other work at the physician-headed Maryland Department of Health (Brunyate & Phelps, 1950). She stated:

> I stayed with Phelps for 21 years. I always took care of Dr. Phelps' home when he was away for the summertime and threw dinners for doctors. There were five men in the United States that were paying any attention to cerebral palsy, and Phelps was the leader; he was "the" man. Phelps asked me to do lectures with his doctors and his therapists.
>
> Later at the Maryland Department of Health and Mental Hygiene, the Secretary of Health and Mental Hygiene, a physician, gave us privileges. We division chiefs sat in on his staffing critique of proposed legislation and his determination of what posture the Health Department was going to take. (Wiemer/Peters oral history, March 18–19, 2003, lines 690–712; 788–791; 879–887; 1,167–1,221; 6,272–6,290)

Fidler remembered psychiatrist Noyes' reputation, recalling:

> Alfred Noyes was one of the authorities who co-authored "the" psychiatric textbook for medical students. I worked in a hospital where Noyes was the superintendent in Pennsylvania. He was a remarkable person. He was such a joy and I learned so much from him. We established a really wonderful relationship. I sent him a copy of the 'OT in Psychiatry' newsletter that I wrote with Betty Ridgway. I have his reply, which says congratulations; this is one of the most insightful pieces of material I have seen. I'm very proud and pleased about that letter. (Fidler/Peters oral history, March 6–7, 2003, lines 316–344)

Yerxa shared her memories about Vernon Nickel, MD at Rancho Los Amigos, saying:

> Dr. Vernon Nickel was the clinical director and he was dynamic, a visionary and a character. He was a great big guy, probably about 6'6", and he looked like Phil Silvers with a baldhead and booming voice. He was a charismatic leader, confrontive and very authoritarian. He was very challenge oriented; you had to know your stuff well enough not to use notes. He had a poster in his office that said let's cut through the soft tissue and get to the bone. He believed PTs [physical therapists] and OTs [occupational therapists] should have maximum autonomy. He said the prescription was chivalrous, and he fostered professional competence. (Yerxa/Peters oral history, April 21–22, 2003, lines 1,564–1,600; 1,612–1,688)

Occupational therapists also believed that co-publishing with physicians lent credibility with a larger audience. Fidler and Llorens talked about their experience in the 1950s and 1960s. Fidler stated, about her 1950 book:

> When I wrote the first book, I knew that it would not be given the time of day unless it had some attachments with credibility. That was when I

seduced my husband [psychiatrist Jay Fidler] into coauthoring. When his name was attached, then it made sense and psychiatrists read it. I had an agenda; if I had to have resorted to other means, I would have. We were real partners in his support of me and the development of OT. (Fidler/ Peters oral history, March 6–7, 2003, lines 212–229; 5,642–5,645)

This Fidler passage illustrates how some community members furthered their professional career through private connections (Fidler, 1984; Fidler & Fidler, 1963). Was Dr. Jay Fidler's commitment to occupational therapy based upon occupational therapy's merits, or his devotion to his wife? Community members Crampton and Llorens spoke highly of Dr. Jay Fidler's psychiatric expert knowledge, and occupational therapy support. However, would he have been such an advocate without the connection to his wife?

Llorens expressed her thinking about physician co-authorship in the 1960s, stating:

Having an MD co-author gave more credibility than if it was just published by me, who was nobody at the time. Medicine carried a lot of weight in all our relationships, even at the national level. It wasn't just a political ploy; I felt they deserved some credit for what they did. It wasn't just what I did that made a difference. After all, they did permit me to do what I did with their patients. They could have said no, you can't do that. (Llorens/Peters oral history, April 25–26, 2003, lines 984–1,007)

Llorens remarks show her gratitude, and at the same time acknowledge that physicians led the treatment team, and made the final patient decisions.

Understandably, introducing occupational therapy to a larger reading audience outside the profession made it better known. What price, however, did occupational therapists have to pay for these alliances? Friedland (1998) argues that occupational therapy forfeited its prevention focus to support medicine's pathology model. The community of therapist insiders considered this a compromise, since it represented a small loss for occupational therapy compared to the professional clout and funding it gained. There were situations when not all therapist and physician alliances proved positive. For example, Welles remembered:

We were respected by physicians if we made it so. We couldn't expect them to respect us. They didn't know what occupational therapy was all about if they just saw patients knitting. I've seen physicians pick up patients' OT activities and throw it all on the floor. They would have to examine the patient, and quickly step out of the room. But I was a great believer in teaching residents and physicians, and having open houses. That's how you did it, by educating. If a physician wanted something made or repaired, we reluctantly did it. But with considerable effort to educate him in the process, and it worked. (Welles/Peters oral history, April 28–29, 2003, lines 3,990–4,025)

Welles described an occupational therapy strength, or back-door approach to power, one that comes from therapist's patience and willingness to educate. If such hospital incidents were indicative of medicine/occupational therapy relationships in the late 1940s, in the 1950s occupational therapists and physical medicine physicians clashed. Physical medicine physicians initially attempted to take over occupational therapy's educational system; however, leaders like Wade and Willard joined forces to maintain independence (West, 1992). Wiemer, a Willard student, stated:

> Helen Willard and Bea Wade had been the ringleaders in breaking us away from physical medicine. In the early days, Helen, for instance was very close to medicine. But that was just the custom, and we went along with it. (Wiemer/Peters oral history, March 18–19, 2003, lines 5,417–5,422)

Bing, a Wade student at the time, explained the physical medicine dilemma, saying:

> The problem with physical medicine was still going on when I was in school at the University of Illinois, College of Medicine at Chicago in the 1950s, but Miss Wade never talked about it. Military hospitals hired these physiatrists and placed OTs and PTs under them. By the end of the war in 1945, physical medicine thought it had earned its specialty within medicine, but could not get recognition. It was not until 1949 when they finally achieved specialty status and that was when they started the big grab for OT and PT. (Bing/Peters oral history, February 6, 2003, lines 29–33 and February 11, 2003, lines 129–148)

Cromwell saw physical therapy's concession stronger than Bing, stating:

> PT lost that battle; they gave up being RPT [registered physical therapist]. They had their own registration but PT caved in because the doctors wanted to take them over and control their certification, so they went to state licensing exclusively. (Cromwell/Peters oral history, April 28–29, 2003, lines 4,948–4,951)

Fearing a similar outcome, occupational therapists remained vigilant, and through omission, or acting like a "poor cousin" to physical therapy in the rehabilitation movement, occupational therapy leaders were able to hold onto independence.

Adding to physiatrists domination, Wiemer[68] looking at physical therapy's experiences, feared that state licensing for occupational therapists would undermine national unity and AOTA's strength and remembered her mid-1960s AOTA presidential concerns, recalling:

> The registration exam was under our aegis. PT's was under medicine for a long time. So our posture was no, lets hang onto registration. Part of my

thinking at the time was that our state groups were not part of the national organization. In physical therapy they are, and this makes a big difference. (Wiemer/Peters oral history, March 18–19, 2003, lines 4,901–4,909)

Secondly, physical therapy, an external agent to this dispute, potentially muddied the picture. In the early 1950s a bill promoting physical therapy licensure in Connecticut stated physical medicine consisted of physical and occupational therapy. AOTA leaders, interpreting this definition as an invitation for physical medicine dominance and a loss of control, officially opposed licensure, resulting in the bill's withdrawal (Gritzer & Arluke, 1985). Cautious and controversial, it took occupational therapy another 20 years to accept state licensure. Cromwell explained the thinking at the time and how occupational therapy remained independent, quietly slipping through the cracks, by stating:

The PTs went to state licensing exclusively after losing their RPT, and they wanted us to do the same. The PTs said the docs don't know beans about what makes a good physical therapist. And we said, they don't even know what OT is. (Cromwell/Peters oral history, April 28–29, 2003, lines 4,955–4,960)

AOTA leaders didn't document the 1940s strife between physical medicine and occupational therapy in official minutes until 1950, thus keeping the debate private from the membership. Establishing a curious precedent, leaders filtered information to the larger membership when handling sensitive issues like licensure and whether occupational therapy was part of Medicare or not 20 years later. Fidler reported that 1970s AOTA leaders believed that Medicare and licensure had the potential to reopen takeover talks that physical medicine introduced in the late 1940s (Fidler/Peters oral history, March 6–7, 2003, lines 2,058–2,065). Thinking of the mid 1960s, Cromwell talked about Medicare, saying:

Medicare was 65. There were more and more regulations laid on top of the health care environment for Medicare coverage. That's when they began defining in the regulations who was an OT or a PT. We had to define who we felt an OT was and the difference between an OTR and a COTA and funding. This carried into the 1970s and 1990s, and now my God, for the last 20 years they're still fighting about what is covered. (Cromwell/Peters oral history April 28–29, 2003, lines 1,484–1,501)

Medicare and licensure remained AOTA hot topics (Cromwell, 1972a, 1972b, 1972c, 1973b, 1973c, 1973d, 1979a, 1979b). For example, AOTA's 1968 Report of the Legislation Committee chaired by Beatrice Wade, with Brunyate Wiemer as a member, showed that Medicare included exploring how occupational therapists could serve directly without a physician's referral and also licensure agenda items (AOTA, October 20, 1968, Council on Development Minutes Annual Conference, Report of Legislation Committee to Council on Development, Addendum 2, Portland Hilton, Portland, Oregon, 9:00 AM–12:00 PM, Crampton private collection).

There was internal division, with a potential to undermine a trajectory toward professionalization. The larger membership did not understand or agree with occupational therapy leaders about physical medicine's actions, thinking any separation from medicine was premature (Colman, 1992; West, 1992). Lacking in West and Colman's accounts of physical medicine's takeover attempt is an analysis of jurisdictional wars. Why in the 1950s, when women had limited professional clout, did occupational therapy win this round of jurisdiction against male-dominated physical medicine? Bing's account however explains that there was internal disagreement in occupational therapy that thwarted any public victory celebration. Bing explained:

> It was some time after graduation that I learned the story and even years later before I got around to asking Bea Wade about it. I point blank asked her why it was so hush-hush, particularly since they won. Bea's response was that there was a lot of disagreement within the political mechanism called AOTA about how it was handled and she and her supporters were roundly criticized for being divisive. Actually, she had saved us our profession, but there were those who felt we should be more polite and ladylike when it comes to MDs. The very idea of a small group of OTs taking on the almighty physicians (physical medicine) was downright godlessness. So, the one thing they all agreed to was to keep their mouths shut, thereby not offending anyone or getting into trouble with any other medical specialty. (Bing/Peters oral history, February 6, 2003, lines 37–49)

AOTA's authority prevailed in 1954 against physical medicine, resulting in occupational therapy's right to develop occupational therapy's educational standards (West, 1992). This guarded victory was misleading because the American Medical Association (AMA) continued to dominate occupational therapy's academic accreditation process until 1980. Cromwell remembers continued challenges during her AOTA presidency from 1967 until 1970. She stated:

> We fought to get out from the AMA (American Medical Association) like we fought the battle with physical medicine who were trying to take us over. I remember going to some of the AMA meetings. Ginny Kilburn was very much admired and praised for what she had done in the preservation of educational standards and got awards from AMA. But I think there were more of us who got to think why are we dependent on physicians for our survival? We better get our own accrediting, and not be in joint accreditation with AMA. We had to be responsible for ourselves and

we had to do our job well. (Cromwell/Peters oral history, April 28–29, 2003, lines 8,207–8,251)

Kilburn represented the old-guard insider view that believed a medical alliance meant respect in the system of professions. In contrast, Cromwell argued for a separation from medicine, reflecting a new point of view that younger therapists like Cromwell and Yerxa proposed.

Occupational therapists, learning from the physical medicine dispute, sought new practice opportunities away from exclusive physician-dominated hospital work. By the 1960s and moving into the 1970s, occupational therapists worked in community mental health centers, some opening their own practices. Federal laws such as the Community Mental Health Centers Act (Public Law 88-164), signed October 31, 1963, just before President Kennedy's death, and staffed under his successor Johnson, opened community mental health work sites to occupational therapists (Bloom, 1977). Slagle recipient therapists such as Gail Fidler, Geraldine Finn, Jerry Johnson, Lela Llorens, and June Sokolov made a mark in this new frontier. Bing remembered the late 1950s/early 1960s shift, stating: "By the end of the decade we began to see a shift from institutionalizing the mentally ill to moving them into the community with mental health centers dotted around the landscape." (Bing/Peters oral history, February 6, 2003, line 80).

On a national level, soon-to-be AOTA president Jerry Johnson, chaired an AOTA committee that wrote a paper recommending the successful integration of occupational therapy with the social and health care systems in the changing decade. Then AOTA President Cromwell remembered the environment that supported this which used more of a systems approach, saying:

That was about the time that Willie (West) went into HEW (Health Education and Welfare), and the Children's Bureau funding started. She helped programs grow. Academic institutions like Boston University, where Jerry was occupational therapy chair, researched and studied things that were affecting children. (Cromwell/Peters oral history, April 28–29, 2003, lines 5,437–5,446)

Continuing this community shift, Cromwell remembered Jerry Johnson's AOTA presidential platform in the early 1970s: "Johnson was very strong on moving into the community and not many had done that yet. We didn't have programs that strongly proposed educational standards. (Cromwell/Peters oral history, April 28–29, 2003, lines 7,013–7,017)

Community mental health was not the only frontier that therapists explored. Occupational therapists entered the public school system when the Johnson Administration's Public Law 94-142 was signed in 1975 and mainstreamed disabled children into regular classrooms.[69] Having far-reaching significance that echoes today, pediatric occupational therapists thus made inroads (Gilfoyle & Hays 1979). Bing remembered how occupational therapy curricula changed as a reaction to Public Law 94-142, recalling:

> In the early 70 s I kept hearing that public education was under fire because kids with disabilities were being educated in poor environments. Parents were beginning to raise questions about "mainstreaming." It occurred to us that we needed to get ready for a shift in practice. In the mid-70s Public Law 94-142 came into being: Education for All Handicapped Children. We had difficulty with the OT students learning the jargon and the public school system. I was very excited about this development because it demonstrated we could coexist in almost any environment. (Bing/Peters oral history, February 29, 2003, lines 998–1,011)

Gilfoyle explained how working on PL 94-142 helped shape her leadership and vision, saying:

> I think about the things that I learned being president of AOTA, and secretary of AOTA, like going out into the public and helping write PL 94-142. I think in terms of my profession, I believe OT allows the empowerment of people. (Gilfoyle/Peters oral history, February 10–11, 2003, lines 1,018–1,028)

Bing, at the University of Texas, Galveston, developed the Rio Grande River Project in 1972, a community program that served underserved families in southern Texas. He explained the 1972–1978 grant funded project and occupational therapy's role in the community, stating:

> We selected Hidalgo, a community right on the Rio Grande River and adopted it since it had no health care providers. The PTs met the high school sports teams and taught them injury prevention. The OTs scattered in the early grades and taught self-worth. We were able to create 7 jobs for OT in the Rio Grande Valley. (Bing/Peters oral history, February 28, 2003, lines 1,012–1,045)

Rooted in a 1960s consciousness, empowerment and equal opportunities were promoted as available for all citizens. The 1960s and 1970s national changes and progressivism stirred the more traditional and conservative 1950s occupational therapy. Occupational therapy leaders questioned professional identity, female roles, education, and diversity (Johnson et al., 1972). Yerxa saw the changing 1960s and 1970s influencing occupational therapy's developing knowledge. She explained:

> The way that we go about articulating and developing our knowledge base is directed by our perceptions as women. It isn't a cold objective scientific approach. Our perceptions, whether it's as women or men, or our particular profession, help us focus on what we think is important.

It has definitely influenced our enculturation and identity. (Yerxa/Peters oral history, April 21–22, 2003, lines 2,089–2,107)

Finding new, more independent roles in the community, occupational therapists revisited questions about autonomy. Discovering new situations outside of hospital settings, therapists began questioning their status as independent professionals.

Professional Identity

Discussions prevalent in the 1970s, about whether occupational therapy was a "true" rather than an emerging profession, brought to light occupational therapy as a predominantly female profession (Fidler, 1977; West, 1992; Yerxa, 1983). Occupational therapy's "charitable ladies" image, stemming from the founding years, did not serve it well in the rehabilitation movement which was indoctrinated with the values of scientific medical environments. On the national front, although America's "golden age" of science spanned World War II to the race to space in the 1960s and 1970s, women scientists experienced a dark period during that time (Rossiter, 1995).[70] This inconsistency affected occupational therapists working in research-oriented clinical settings or universities.

Identifying as "second class" and characterizing occupational therapy as an acquiescent "feminine" profession was counterproductive (Yerxa, 1975). Seemingly the 1960s women's movement minimally influenced occupational therapists, with few conversations at their places of employment or professional conferences.[71] Leaders argued for more professional autonomy and the need for assertive occupational therapy practitioners (Cromwell, 1970a; Fidler, 1977, 1979a; Yerxa, 1967b, 1975, 1978, 1979, 1980, 1982, 1983a, 1983b, 1983c, 1986). Occupational therapists needed not only be autonomous but committed to the profession; 34% of AOTA members stopped working after 10 years of practice to raise families (Jantzen, 1972a, 1972b; Mathewson, 1975). Similarly, many nurses entered their careers anticipating leaving when they become mothers, unless economic demands required continued work (Simpson & Simpson, 1969). One drawback to this pattern is that work discontinuation led women to be in a poor competitive position with men.[72] Bing remembered the 1950s occupational therapy workforce shortage related to career interruptions, stating:

The real problem in the 50s was the fact that a typical OT practiced an average of 3 to 4 years, then disappeared, usually into marriage. The schools could not turn out enough additional people to cover this loss. As I recall there were only about 4,000 OTs when I came in, in 1952. A decade later it was not too much better. Additionally, there was a very slow growth of new schools. (Bing/Peters oral history, February 11, 2003, lines 218–223)

Men's work shaped the family financially, by class, privilege, and location. Women experienced an unresolved tension between family life and individual goals (Degler, 1980). This argument is well-supported in the 1950s traditional two-parent household, but weakens in the context of non-traditional family structures, as societal values changed in the 1960s. Predominantly female, occupational therapists experienced societal tensions and dilemmas that many professional women experienced. Marketplace work did not take precedence (Coontz, 2000; Rosenow, 1982). Typically, women continued to work around family needs first, placing them in a weaker economic position than working men (Fuchs, 1988). Secondly, women experienced stress when balancing roles including wife, mother, homemaker, and worker with limited time.[73] Third, some therapists left disenchanted with occupational therapy. Wiemer remembers a Maryland occupational therapist who left the profession. She recalls:

> When I was president in 1964 there was a woman whom I considered bright, and she was one of these disenchanted OTs who married an afflu-ent man and didn't have to work. I went to her and said, can I come to you once in a while and just chew the apple? We talked a good deal about how OT should focus itself in order to stay firm and strong. She was disenchanted with the arts and crafts as entertainment image. (Wiemer/Peters oral history, March 18–19, 2003, lines 3,056–3,080)

Fourth, there was an additional concern that occupational therapists who sought their graduate education in other disciplines would leave the profession, potentially draining a pool of scholars. Bing and Yerxa remem-bered this at the doctoral level. Bing talked about being the seventh therapist nationwide to earn a doctorate in 1961, saying:

> I met with considerable resistance inside OT; many thought I was getting too big for my britches and that I was seeking a way out of OT. They sim-ply could not understand why anyone in OT would want a doctoral degree. (Bing/Peters oral history, February 11, 2003, lines 267–270)

Yerxa supported Bing's perception that doctorates in other fields could mean an exit in the 1960s, stating:

> There was a concern that people who had been trained doctorally in other fields would then be snapped up and exit, even though they had been financially supported by these grants. I don't think that happened very much. I think OTs are so committed. When I was the research coordinator at Rancho I had an appointment in the School of Medicine (University of Southern California), and I think they would have liked to have me come there on a more full-time basis, but I wasn't interested. I wasn't interested in anything but getting back to OT. (Yerxa/Peters oral history, April 21–22, 2003, lines 2,536–2,544)

Yerxa remembered therapists thinking about developing occupational therapy doctoral education, relaying:

> I think in the 1960s there were some people thinking about a doctorate in occupational therapy. Certainly Anne Mosey was and Wilma West thought in the future we needed to have doctoral level education in OT. It was just a dream at that point. (Yerxa/Peters oral history April 21–22, 2003, lines 2,489–2,543)

Career-minded occupational therapists in the 1960s sought graduate education while juggling family responsibilities, including child care or taking care of elderly parents (Gilligan Kapcar, 1976). For example Wiemer, juggling her full-time senior position at the Maryland Department of Health and Hygiene while managing family financial affairs involving her mother and brother, remembered earning her master's degree at Johns Hopkins University in 1967. She recalled:

> When I went for my master's I asked for funds because my counterpart in PT got full financial support. He was getting his degree in public health. The business administration would not give me a nickel because I was getting mine in education. I was responsible at that time for the OT assistant's curriculum, which was freestanding under the Maryland Department of Health and Mental Hygiene. Bill, the PT, got a leave of absence to do his public health degree, I didn't. Thanks to my supervisor, Dr. Jean Ruth Stickler, who saw me drag out the degree, said I wouldn't even know if you're not here, and she gave me time to really finish it. (Wiemer/Peters oral history, March 18–19, 2003, lines 1,596–1,618)

Wiemer balanced her limited time between her job responsibilities, and family responsibilities. Gender discrimination affected her during the more open minded 1960s. Wiemer noted other gender imbalances in her administrative job and saw a need for workplace equality. She discussed how occupational therapy was overlooked because of its characteristic feminine traits, stating: "In the 60 s there were very few women in administrative jobs, or who had any introduction to business administration or economics. Most of us came out of liberal arts, the arts or nursing" (Wiemer/Peters oral history, March 18–19, 2003, lines 5,759–5,762).

Occupational therapists, such as Gilfoyle and Llorens, balanced traditional family lives, taking care of their homes, carpooling children, and meeting career demands. Gilfoyle spoke about moving from full-time work to a more flexible federal grant-funded project when she became a mother, saying:

> I left JFK because we had adopted Sean and I didn't want to work full-time. I had an opportunity to work part-time on a three-year HEW (Health Education and Welfare) child abuse grant at Denver General that later became Denver Health Sciences Center. That was about 1966 or 1967. (Gilfoyle/ Peters February 10–11, 2003, lines 1,327–1,337; 1,374; 1,458)

Llorens balanced her career and family responsibilities creatively with her husband. She explained:

> When we moved to Florida our daughter Maria was in first or second grade. We had a young adult come when she got home from school. That lasted until third grade, and then Joe was teaching at a community college and his hours were flexible. He could be home when she came home from school. I could manage my position and do the mommy things that I wanted to do like go to PTA meetings and parent teacher conferences. I got up at 5:00 in the morning and did an hour or so of writing before I got Maria up. (Llorens/Peters oral history, April 25–26, 2003, lines 1,329–1,350; 2,961–2,977)

Others like Fidler, Wiemer, and Crampton redefined their family roles. Fidler challenged child care traditions, alternating times when she remained at home with times when she traveled distances to consulting positions away from her family. Wiemer and Crampton cared for elderly parents while gaining career achievements. Fidler navigated her career first, spent months at a time away from home, commuting back on weekends. Fidler explained how she balanced her roles as wife and mother with her professional career, saying:

> It was never easy; I struggled all the time with a sense of guilt, you know you just do. I knew what I had to do for me, and I will always remember the time I was home for a while, and my 9-year-old son said to me when are you going back to work? I said, why do you ask? He said because you're a better mother when you work. I had a contract with myself that I had to earn enough money to pay a full-time nanny and housekeeper.
>
> The career moves were mine, not my husband's. I went to AOTA, he was home in New Jersey and I was in Washington. I came home on weekends if I wasn't on the West Coast. My mother didn't understand, and thought it would come to no good-end. She would say every time I would go home to visit, be nice to (husband) Jay. I would say why don't you tell Jay to be nice to me? Talk about gender bias. There wasn't a feminist movement when I started; there just wasn't. I was just out there. (Fidler/ Peters oral history, March 6–7, 2003, lines 3,106–3,120; 3,650–3,716)

Wiemer married later in life, retiring in 1980 and devoting more time to her private life. Cromwell and Welles created a family in their more than 54-year partnership, blending their public occupational therapy lives with their private lives. Bing, Crampton, Stattel, and Yerxa never married. Yerxa remembered messages learned early in her life about role stereotypes and a woman's pursuing a professional career, stating:

> I didn't see any barriers. However, when I was 12 years old I was thinking about becoming a physician. I'm so glad I didn't become a physician

but I remember my mother saying; well, honey, I don't think you really want to do that because you'll want to get married. (Yerxa/Peters oral history, April 21–22, 2003, lines 646–661)

The feminist movement, although sought to increase professional opportunities for women, was not occupational therapy's simple solution, with some supporting the movement and others noting their disinterest. For example, Welles stated; "I'm not very interested in women's roles" (Welles/Peters oral history, April 28–29, 2003, line 3306). Other occupational therapy leaders spoke about their discontent with the feminist movement and its potential undermining influence on occupational therapy. For example, Fidler, progressive in her own career, felt that once opportunities opened in traditionally male-dominated professions because of the equal rights movement, occupational therapy would be left with less qualified women. She stated:

Way back, the women were very bright and had nowhere to go academically. They couldn't enter medicine; the bona fide professions were not open to women. When society changed in the 1960s, and medicine, dentistry, and psychology opened, all these bright women left, and we were left with second string. (Fidler/Peters oral history, March 6–7, 2003, lines 1,483–1,497; 1,575–1,581)

Gilfoyle shared two perspectives about the feminist movement, one supportive, and the other critical. She considered the feminist movement a political shield when occupational therapy programs experienced difficult times. Gilfoyle explained a tenuous situation at Colorado State University, when its occupational therapy program was in jeopardy of closing, saying:

Politically, they weren't going to get rid of a women's profession. It was at the time of the women's movement in the 60s and 70s. To be politically correct you couldn't touch them, and I knew that. Whether I liked it or not, I took advantage of it. (Gilfoyle/Peters oral history, February 10–11, 2003, lines 2,848–2,853)

Although Gilfoyle acknowledged the political safety net that the women's movement may have carried to occupational therapy's workplace, she believed some of her occupational therapy peers took the feminist platform to an extreme and became biased against men unfairly. According to Gilfoyle, these therapists broadened their platform beyond criticizing the stereotypical male physician domination of a feminized occupational therapy profession. This, she thought, actually worked against the female therapist's sense of empowerment. Presenting a fuller picture, Gilfoyle explained that feminism linked to lesbianism introduced another political and sociological layer and complexity in the community of therapists and their perceptions of society. She stated:

> The renaissance of the feminist movement was a shock and disappoint-ment to me in occupational therapy. I could not identify with how angry so many women were about men. We have a lot of lesbians in the pro-fession who were angry. When I look back, they had to hide in the closet. I knew that out there in society the opportunities were a little different, but I always felt equal to men. I believed you're in charge of yourself; you're in charge of where you're going to go. If we're going to change, we're going to change because of us, not because we're changing for men. As a society we have to respect the female culture and male culture, learn the rules of the game, embrace and capitalize on the differences. Respect them, and we'll continue to have opportunities for women. (Gilfoyle/Peters oral history, February 10–11, 2003, lines 1,827–1,887; 1,965–1,968)

Disagreeing, Llorens did not see the alleged sexual orientation-driven anger that Gilfoyle sensed, rather the predominant view that therapists didn't like the confines of the male-dominated medical system. She stated:

> I don't think I ever associated the negativity towards the medical model as related to a person's sexual orientation. I did see some people where the negativity related to the male medical model as a reaction against male domination, but I saw that among heterosexual and potentially homosexual people. I think it was a matter of having built a profession and feeling that it still was not accepted enough. (Llorens/Peters oral history April 25–26, 2003, lines 5,306–5,320)

Fidler reported sensitivity to any male symbolism in a predominantly female profession. She took issue with AOTA's honorary title inaugurated in 1973, Fellow of the American Occupational Therapy Association (FAOTA), that most community members earned, stating:

> I was in the first group; I objected strongly to calling us fellows. In a woman's organization you aren't a fellow. It's because of medicine. Nursing doesn't have fellows; they're smarter than we are. Oh, I was disgusted! (Fidler/Peters oral history, March 6–7, 2003, lines 6,652–6,676)

Not only gender issues influenced the community of therapists' actions; society was changing. Yerxa earning her doctoral degree at Boston University in the 1960s and remembered Boston's social climate, by saying:

> There is an incongruity in my thinking between my Slagle writings and my doctoral studies thinking. I don't think it dawned on me until I

really started to get into my doctoral study and the world of the 60 s, which was so dramatic in Boston. It was the time when Martin Luther King was assassinated and the students at Kent State killed. I was a TA [teaching assistant] and many of my classes were canceled because of bomb scares; students were taking over the administration building. I was a TA in Ed Psych [Education Psychology], and the students took over my class. It was an unbelievable experience. I wouldn't change it for anything. (Yerxa/Peters oral history, April 21–22, 2003, lines 2,206–2,220)

Responding to a changing society, the occupational therapy class, gender, and racial mix began changing, although minimally. No longer were occupational therapy student applicants accepted from the private tony or exclusive women's schools as in the 1930s and 1940s. The Suzy Slagle ranks diversified as the working middle class, and lower-middle class therapists earned their degrees at state universities like Llorens, a Western Michigan State University graduate.[74]

Llorens broke racial barriers in her esteemed career. Speaking candidly about the 1970s in racially segregated Florida, she said about her University of Florida, Gainesville faculty appointment: "At the time it was politically correct to have a woman, a Black and a Catholic, and I fit all three" (Llorens/Peters oral history, April 25–26, 2003, lines 2,182–2,183).

Experiencing racial tensions as a Student Affiliation Council delegate to the AOTA national conference in New Orleans, Louisiana in 1961, Llorens spoke about the institutional racism that prevented her from attending the meeting. Louisiana, maintaining a racial separatist policy, had prevented Whites and African Americans to associate. Responding to the situation, AOTA went on record and established an anti-discrimination policy. She explained:

The first meeting that I was to attend at the national level was being held in New Orleans. New Orleans was segregated in 1961. It turned out that I could not attend the meeting because I couldn't sit in the same room with my colleagues because there was a state statute that said Black people and White people couldn't be associated. Before I learned about the statute, I heard I couldn't stay at the hotel. I said fine, I'd stay at the Y, and bring a peanut butter and jelly sandwich in a brown paper bag. When Lyla Spelbring, who had a position with AOTA related to the Student Affiliation Council, found out I couldn't sit in the room, she had a fit. AOTA went on record immediately that they would not have any meetings booked at any hotels that discriminated against any members. It wasn't their fault; I was the first person this happened to. They didn't have any other African American people who were representatives or who were officers at the national level. That was my first national position. (Llorens/Peters oral history, April 25–26, 2003, lines 1,214–1,265; 5,012–5,035)

In a fascinating twist of events, Llorens, in 1969 presenting her Slagle lecture in front of 1,000 members of AOTA remembered what the experience was like in Dallas, Texas, saying:

> We stayed in the hotel; nobody was mean to us or showed us problems. The breathtaking part of it happened when I arrived at the huge auditorium. It was filled primarily with white women. On the balcony, it was ringed with cooks, bellhops, and maids, Black people who worked in the hotel. They were standing and listening to my lecture. The word had spread that this Black woman was up there talking to these women, and they were there to hear and probably lend support.
>
> Ruth Whipple Pershing, a classmate of mine at Western Michigan was the first Dean of the School of Occupational Therapy at Texas Woman's University. After the lecture, she had seven or eight African American students, whom she brought up on stage. They were so proud; it was very wonderful. (Llorens/Peters oral history, April 25–26, 2003, lines 2,304–2,337)

In that same vein, Llorens accepted a White House invitation in 1970, as a California delegate to a Children and Youth Conference. She remembered this non occupational therapy event, saying:

> I was very flattered to be invited. Dr. Ruth Gross was the Children and Youth Project Chairperson, and Wilma West was the sponsor of the Children and Youth projects nationally. The conference was planned to get people together to lay out a 10-year program for children and youth and the ideas were going to be grist for the legislative mill. (Llorens/ Peters oral history, April 25–26, 2003, lines 4,883–4,906)

As a leader and scholar, Llorens supported a unified profession, not one delimited by socioeconomic or racial divisions. This is seen in her involvement in AOTA's Black Caucus, a group that formed in 1975. She explained the group's purpose and structure, stating:

> I was involved with the Black Caucus from the very beginning. The idea was to have a place and time where Black occupational therapists and students could get together to talk about issues. Later some mentoring occurred. There was an issue about whether the meeting should be open or closed. I was one of the vocal people who said it could not be closed. And while people honored the fact that Black therapists wanted to get together and not storm the gates, my reasoning was if there were any other meetings that were closed and Blacks couldn't go to them, they'd be screaming. The meetings were always open; you don't close the whole meeting to other people who are in the same profession as you. (Llorens/Peters oral history, April 25–226, 2003, lines 5,162–5,193)

This underlying, unifying belief that Llorens expressed, was the same belief system that the community of therapists shared when they promoted occupational therapy externally.

This section explored how occupational therapy leaders navigated the profession within a larger social system. It discussed how a cadre of predominantly female therapists used covert strategies to gain authority and autonomy in a predominantly male medical environment amongst physicians and other health care professionals. Participating in the rehabilitation movement, feminist movement, and equality movements resulted in setting up a chain of events where therapists entered new arenas, addressed professional identity and began to accept a more diversified membership. In the final section, I discuss an overview, and place occupational therapy's history in a more current context.

SECTION VIII: OCCUPATIONAL THERAPY'S PAST INFLUENCES ITS PRESENT, AND CONCLUSION

Occupational therapy's past and present are bridged in a common goal. That is, developing occupational therapy's knowledge base was and is a professional priority, to better understand the outcomes of practice, and for occupational therapy's viability (AOTA & AOTF, 2004; AOTF, 1975; Llorens & Gillette, 1985). Understanding how occupational therapy's past influences the profession today, can be explored by asking two questions. First, what can we learn from those who created and supported occupational therapy's science-based knowledge from the 1950s until 1980? Secondly, what significance does knowledge development have in better understanding how professions develop autonomy in a larger historical and sociological context?

By forming a community of therapists, the occupational therapy scholars and leaders involved in knowledge development, changed occupational therapy,by bridging the gap between practice and theory and making occupational therapy known to society. Their legacy was their belief in occupational therapy and knowing that professionalization meant not only developing a scientific body of knowledge, but also finding the right opportunities, people, and liaisons to better position occupational therapy in the health care and educational systems. In so doing, occupational therapy entered a system of professions, setting up a chain of events that ultimately led to occupational therapy's professionalism, and autonomy from almost 50 years of male physician domination.

The community's story is an account of how and why a small group of occupational therapy scholars and leaders created a community by association and their contributions that helped their profession expand and thrive. This community lacked homogeneity, and had insiders and outsiders. Community entrance came from educational pedigree, or introduction and mentorship. Primarily, this was a group of powerful women, working in clinical, academic, and administrative roles who knew each other's strengths and weaknesses. Building occupational therapy together, community insiders gave countless volunteer hours, and their own monies when needed to expand AOTA and AOTF. Community outsiders, or occupational therapy scholars and leaders who developed theories and expanded a scientific knowledge base, held dissimilar views from the leadership mainstream. They challenged occupational therapy's traditional views and introduced new thinking to the profession.

Riding the crest of the waves from the country's 1960s science preoccupation and the women's movement, these women entered surroundings previously unfamiliar to a majority of occupational therapists, like legislative lobbying, federal and state health care positions, and academic administration. Discovered in each of their stories is their connection to Wilma West, who led the profession and the community through grit, determination and financial skill. Leading a single-minded group of professionals when addressing occupational therapy's worth, the community of therapists fought for and gained autonomy and credibility as a bona fide profession by articulating what they did, establishing rationales behind their work, and foretelling its projected outcomes to benefit society.

Finding their own voice through scholarship and leadership, occupational therapists responded to social and historical events influencing this country that strengthened their resolve to move the profession forward. Yerxa, summarizing her thinking, stated:

> One of the things that has really struck me is how we are all influenced by our times, and by our context. The depression, World War II, the 60 s and post modernism have all had a great influence on me. A strong part of it is the history of the status of women. That too is imbedded in my career. I see the profession having achieved much more autonomy in my lifetime than I probably ever would have dreamed, going back to the old days of the medical prescription. I think it's been a hard struggle, but we have been able to be set free though our own thinking from medicine. We offer important contributions to human life. (Yerxa/Peters oral history, April 21–22, 2003, lines 4,696–4,727)

Therapists negotiated occupational therapy's place in the rehabilitation, equal rights, and feminist movement during the 1950s up until 1980. Community members known in their work environments and through publications, established occupational therapy's place amongst other professions. Internally, the community of therapists were the leaders, decision makers, and intellectual authorities who the larger professional membership knew by name or reputation. Trusting each other, community members kept certain information private, like physical medicine's potential takeover or sealing the Slagle meeting tapes. Did these decisions that set leaders apart from the larger membership establish an internal separateness, an occupational therapy class system or a stratification like that in any human association? These matters, although red-flagged to a student of history, may have gone unnoticed or have been of little concern to the typical occupational therapist.

Perhaps the potential separation between the community of therapists and the larger membership is a problem in itself. What did the larger membership know or care about occupational therapy frames of references or research development? To their credit, the community of therapists facilitated avenues for all occupational therapists to be involved in such lofty goals, through organizational restructuring that separated AOTA and created a new think tank in AOTF. Secondly, the Delegate Assembly reorganization and renaming to become the Representative Assembly may have permitted more grass roots involvement. Finally, setting aside annual monies from AOTA membership fees that supported the foundation's mission meant that every occupational therapist had a vested interest in occupational therapy's knowledge development.

This was a dynamic 30-year period in occupational therapy's history that marked the development of a new professional culture. Gilfoyle believed that changing occupational therapy's culture required perceptions that she described as a political maneuver when saying:

> It takes changing the critical mass of a culture or 10% to 15% of the people over 30 years for things to change, in 10-year increments. For example, when I was at AOTA there were around 4,000 members, and if we could bring along 400 people we could change the profession. I think we're right in the middle of changing some of our cultural theories in the profession, it's evolving. (Gilfoyle/Peters oral history, February 10–11, 2003, lines 1,704–1,731)

Gilfoyle's 30-year change analysis echoes my own view that occupational therapy gained its professional authority over three decades, in 10-year increments.

Occupational therapy's more conservative 1950s saw therapists functioning under doctors' prescriptions, and therapists' names followed physicians' names in publications. The more radical 1960s women questioned their roles, and therapists questioned physician domination and why occupational therapy worked. Theory development efforts as well as independent authorships and political activism characterized the 1970s. The 1970s marked a more formal knowledge organization, with leaders debating about scientific and philosophical differences, and learned about research in graduate education, continuing education workshops, and seminars.

Synthesizing this study, and by capturing their words, there was an overwhelming feeling that occupational therapy not only brought meaning to those it served but to the leaders and scholars who dedicated their careers to its betterment. Welles, stated simply; "I'm glad I found OT. I hope it persists" (line 4628). Yerxa identified the profession as seductive and baffling, saying:

> This profession is extremely seductive, and most challenging. It's so hard to grasp, but that's what makes it fascinating, because I've always felt it isn't finished yet. It's still developing and we have the potential to change society. Our future can be shaped by how we can identify our science. (Yerxa/Peters oral history, April 21–22, 2003, lines 2,548–2,593; 4,886–4,888; 4,895–4,900)

If, in fact, a community of therapists were occupational therapy's change agents 50-years ago, will a similar group continue to shape their work?

Does a current community continue the debate about scientific inquiry where this community left off, and do they borrow strategies for change, studying occupational therapy's place in the larger system of professions? Specifically, like the community of therapists, do current leaders and scholars look to society's changes, with an eye to historical implications in future years? As occupational therapist ranks grow, does the number of practicing therapists have an effect on how change takes place? Martha Kirkland, Executive Director AOTF, with an eye to the future stated:

> I think while we do need to document our effectiveness and efficacy in the current health care environment, if we focus on just that, we're going to be out of business in five years when the environment changes. You can't move out if you look only at today. We are quite free to move beyond and look at different models of practice. Looking at OT's role today, and 5 years or 10 years from now, is being able to look at trends out of the box. (Kirkland/Peters interview, March 21, 2003, lines 1,214–1,248)

Perhaps the current debate about basic and applied scientific inquiry remains too narrow when defining occupational therapy's future path. I argue that knowledge type and focus does not make or break a profession, for at occupational therapy's heart are the people who guarded and invested their ideas and foresight. The community of therapists discovered that knowledge alone was not enough to make occupational viable. Rather, their stories dealt with power, at a time when women professionals were not seen as dynamic change agents. They exhibited their power differently, either politically, intellectually, or through persistence, all believed in occupational therapy's worth. Fifty years ahead of its time, this community looked beyond their daily routines to reshape the profession.

Conclusion

In conclusion, this work illustrated how a community of therapists negotiated occupational therapy's professional power and place in the rehabilitation, equal rights, and feminist movements during the 1950s until 1980. This however remains an isolated and perhaps one-sided story if I didn't ask what could those outside of occupational therapy learn from this particular case study about professional development? Specifically, what contributions can occupational therapy make to oral history, the history of professions, and women's history?

Oral history, gaining strides from the 1960s equal rights movement, typically captured the stories of the disenfranchised lower class or "invisible" Americans who did not have professional title or socio-economic power. Oral history made these people known by creating a historical record about their lives. In contrast, the people I studied using oral history were "visible" Americans. Known in their profession, they came from middle and advantaged upper-middle class backgrounds.

Secondly, these scholars and leaders left documents and publications, or a paper trail that could be studied and analyzed. Adding to their published works, I had the opportunity to directly question the authors about the context and meaning, which enabled me to understand historical circumstances prior to making any interpretations. Hence oral history became a more objective source of inquiry than if the print documents stood alone. Unique in this work is how oral histories challenged, expanded, and in the case of sealed documents, told a deeper and more telling story. Therefore, I argue there is a strong need for using oral history in conjunction with print sources. There is also a need to use oral history with all people, expanding it beyond the disenfranchised, to include a more public people, to better understand why these decision makers chose different paths in the context of their times.

Expanding the literature about history of professions, and women's history, occupational therapy as a female dominated profession did not collapse or subsume to more dominant professions like physical medicine. Understanding how the community of therapists remained "ladylike" while doing "unladylike" things teaches the reader lessons about professional evolution and turf wars. Using charm and intellect, this capable community of therapists used power to professionalize. Wearing their pearls, hats, and gloves these post-1950s women forged razor tuff negotiations over martinis in smoke filled rooms behind political doors. Rather than deferring, these women embraced gender inequities using their female networking strategies to overcome challenges. As an enduring test to their actions and documentation of a profession's autonomy, occupational therapy was not marginalized, subsumed or dominated by other professions. Rather than becoming male-like or medicine-like, this female dominated profession strategically glorified its feminization as it became scientific, thus providing a unique template to gender specific professions. Therefore occupational therapy's story of struggle, survival, scholarship, and expansion bring much to understanding power and professionalization.

NOTES

1. To reduce conflict, female nursing leaders hoped men would enter the profession and change the gender dominated stereotypes, as well as the usual thinking of the time (Faludi, 1991; Manley, 1995).

2. Historian Reverby has experience studying health care professions which are predominantly female. In 1970, she was working at the Health Policy Advisory Center in New York, where she studied women health workers. (Reverby, 1987, p. xi). This led to her 1987 book, *Ordered to care: The dilemma of American nursing, 1850 to 1945*, Cambridge University Press.

3. Various occupational therapy scholars have written about occupational therapy's knowledge development, including models, frames of reference, or (continued) theoretical conceptualizations of practice (Barris, Kielhofner, & Watts, 1988; Gillette & Kielhofner, 1979; Kielhofner, 1997; Kielhofner & Burke, 1977, 1983;Please confirm change from Kielhofner 1983 to Kielhofner & Burke 1983 in match References. Llorens, 1976; Mosey, 1981, 1985, 1996; Reed & Sanderson, 1999).

4. The "traditional epistemological orientation" to practice is a school of thought using practical information, gathered from observation, reasoning, and trial and error, as a foundation for practice. The "disciplinal epistemological orientation" to practice is a school of thought using a single comprehensive theory, usually developed through basic scientific inquiry, as a foundation for practice. Basic scientific inquiry uses the methods of science to develop accurate theories about the physical universe. The "neopositivistic epistemological orientation" to practice is a school of thought using applied scientific information, primarily in the form of guidelines for practice, developed by applied scientific inquiry, as a foundation for practice. Applied scientific inquiry uses the methods of science and theoretical information to address practical problems. A "phenomenological epistemological orientation" to practice is a school of thought using a case approach that views each person as unique. Phenomenological inquiry uses theoretical postulates, individual case studies, and protocols to address individual problems.

5. Manley's (1995) nursing study employs the System of Professions model. Patients' needs, an external *social force* (highest level), augmented by physicians requesting nursing services, initiated a chain effect at the *system of professions* (middle level of model), where jurisdictional power disputes occurred. Nursing manpower needs led to the *differentiation* (lowest level) process when registered nurses separated from vocationally trained practical nurses.

6. Sociological-behavioral historians use specific models examining how and why a society, movement, or institution developed in a specific place and time (Cantor & Schneider, 1967).

7. Fischer (1970) argues that the goal of historical inquiry is paradigm building based on selected truths, leading to specific conclusions, rather than story reconstruction. Kaestle (1996) believes that historians are tentative when claiming truths about the past because historical truths are relative and plural. For example, several eyewitnesses can view the same event completely differently.

8. The interview framework followed Tuchman's (1981) "elements of historical communication" (pp. 55–60), stating that: (1) something is worth saying; (2) the content is a synthesis of ideas; and (3) the historian uses intuition to better understand past circumstances.

9. Elizabeth (Becky) Engleke Holdeman (1954) authored "Occupational therapy for patients with anterior poliomyelitis," in H. S. Willard & C. S. Spackman (Eds.), *Principles of Occupational Therapy*, 2nd ed., Lippincott, Philadelphia. Stattel refers to Holdeman's position as Director of Occupational Therapy, Veterans Administrative Center, Wadworth General Hospital, Los Angeles, California.

10. Majorie Fish was AOTA Executive Director 1961–1964.

11. Helen Willard was AOTA President 1958–1961.

12. Cordelia Meyers, MA, OTR, started editing the *American Journal of Occupational Therapy* in 1968 during Cromwell's presidency.

13. "Susie Slagle"refers to novelist Augusta Tucker's 1939 book *Miss Susie Slagle's*, Harper and Brothers, New York, that lightheartedly recounts how Miss Slagle's "maternal instincts had gone into culinary channels keeping a medical boarding house" for "doctors in the making" (p. 15) at Johns Hopkins University.

14. Mrs. Greene, although socially established, was not an occupational therapist.

15. In 1963, 389 occupational therapists held graduate degrees, out of 6,105 (constituting 6%). Therapists earning advanced degrees after their occupational therapy requirements more than quadrupled between 1950 (19%) to 1962 (90%). Of those, three earned doctor of philosophy (PhD) degrees, two earned doctor of education (Ed D) degrees, and the rest earned Master's degrees (Jantzen et al., 1964).

16. Fidler earned a Bachelor of Arts Degree in education and psychology, Lebonon Valley College, 1938 and OT Certificate, 1942, Philadelphia School of Occupational Therapy (Ludwig, 1988a).

17. Reilly graduated from Girl's Latin High School in Boston. (Van Deusen, 1988).

18. Reilly, M., Ed. (1974). *Play as Exploratory Learning*. Beverly Hills, CA, Sage Publishing.

19. To provide a career context, Reilly published less than 20 juried articles compared to Llorens' and Ayres' publication record, both of which were around four or five times greater.

20. Fidler and Fine, collaborating since the 1960s, developed a projective occupational therapy mental health evaluation tool, the Object History, in 1970. Unpublished manuscript cited in Ludwig (1988a), p. 31.

21. Yerxa conceptualized occupational science in the late 1980s while formulating an occupational therapy doctorate program. Occupational science was expanded and further developed in the 1990s by University of Southern California occupational therapy faculty, Clark et al., (1991) as an academic discipline using a basic science approach.

22. Johnson, unable to give an oral history because of poor health, was the 1972 Slagel lecturer, 1979 Award of Merit recipient, and AOTA president following Cromwell. Johnson, a futurist supporting social reform at the (continued) grassroots level, often went against traditional occupational therapy views. Community members Bing, Fidler, and Gilfoyle spoke about Johnson's outsider status, and controversial actions. Fidler referred to Johnson as the populist AOTA President. Bing stated: "Johnson was using her place to reinvent and reorganize OT. It caused a great deal of trouble because there were some important people around who had not forgiven her her transgression when she was president in the 70 s. I understand she is quite ill." (Bing/Peters oral history, March 7, 2003, lines 1325–1332).

23. Further identifying in alphabetical order banquet participants, Fish was AOTA executive director 1961–1963, and AOTA Award of Merit recipient, 1964; Gleave was AOTA Award of Merit recipient, 1967; McDaniel was AOTA Award of Merit recipient, 1968; Robinson was AOTA president 1955–1958, and AOTA Award of Merit recipient in 1959; Spackman was AOTA Award of Merit recipient, 1956; Spelbring was AOTA Award of Merit recipient, 1971; Spear was AOTA Award of Merit recipient, 1960; Wiemer, AOTA president 1964–1967, AOTA Slagle lecturer 1957, AOTA Award of Merit, 1968; and Willard was AOTA president 1958–1961, and AOTA Award of Merit recipient, 1954.

24. Jerry Johnson's AOTA Presidency began in 1974.

25. Occupational therapist Mary Fiorentino was the 1974 Eleanor Clarke Slagle lecturer. Fiorentino (1975) paralleled the development of the occupational therapy profession through its body of knowledge, and an occupational therapist's professional development to a child's maturing central nervous system in her lecture "Occupational Therapy: Realization to activation." Fiorentino acknowledged Grady, Gilfoyle, and Moore in her presentation.

26. Duke Kahanamoku, Olympic gold medal swimmer and freestyle record holder in 1912 and 1920, and water polo medalist in 1932, taught the athletic Crampton surfing (International Swimming Hall of Fame, retrieved May 4, 2005 from http://www.ishof.org/65dkahanamoku.html).

27. According to Stattel, New York Senator and Mrs. George Thompson were family friends and neighbors in Kings Park, New York.

28. Stattel was the director of occupational therapy and vocational services at Rehabilitation Shops, sponsored by Connecticut Society for Crippled Children and Adults, Inc., in Bridgeport, Connecticut, from 1945 until 1947. This coincided with her studies at New York University.

29. Stattel received her charter World Federation of Occupational Therapists (WFOT) membership application from Clare Spackman. Spackman, who collected Stattel's $3.00 membership fee was a WFOT treasurer, according to another early WFOT member Cromwell. Cromwell stated; "Clare (Spackman) and Helen (Willard) were very big in WFOT." (Cromwell oral history, August 28–29, 2003, line 2030). Spackman wrote Stattel; "you realize of course that you are our first members," (Spackman to Stattel letter, University of Pennsylvania, December 8, 1952, Stattel private collection).

30. The National Society of The Colonial Dames of America (NSCDA), founded in 1891 and headquartered in Washington D.C., preserves national heritage through museum projects, historical activities including a colonial register, and patriotic service. There are 44 corporate societies with over 15,000 members. Retrieved May 19, 2005 from http://www.nscda.org.

31. The West family farm was located outside of Rochester, New York, near Clifton Springs, New York, occupational therapy's founding location.

32. Kahmann was AOTA's president 1947 to 1952, and Award of Merit recipient in 1952. Robinson was AOTA's president 1955 to 1958, and Award of Merit recipient in 1959. Gleave was AOTA's Award of Merit recipient in 1967. Spackman was AOTA's Award of Merit recipient in 1956. Crampton was AOTA's

Award of Merit recipient in 1972. Kilburn was AOTA's former director of professional education and Award of Merit recipient in 1976.

33. "In the mid-1950s AOTA received monies from two grants. Mary Alice Coombs, who was from the Texas Department of Mental Health and Mental Retardation, felt that her job was to regionalize therapists, so they could form support groups and provide training to up-grade practice." (Bing/Peters oral history, February 12, 2003, lines 205–215).

34. Bing lived with Dunton, 1957 through 1959, at his Baltimore, Maryland home while a full- time doctoral student. Acting as an aide and personal assistant, Bing had full access to Dunton's private papers.

35. Bing was a staff occupational therapist, United States Army, Medical Services, Fitzsimons Army Hospital (FAH), Aurora, Colorado, from 1951 until 1953, and used his GI Bill award for his Master's degree.

36. West referred to a 1979 AOTA Representative Assembly Resolution 537-79 that supported transitioning research responsibilities to AOTF.

37. Spear, a community insider and colleague to academic program directors Wade, Willard, and Fish, received AOTA's Award of Merit in 1960 and graduated from the Boston School of Occupational Therapy.

38. Llorens attended the College of Puget Sound, majoring in occupational therapy, prior to transferring to Western Michigan University. Describing Puget Sound's occupational therapy program director who first admitted her, Llorens said: "Edna Ellen Bell, who was the chair at Puget Sound, was a crusty kind of military veteran, with an 'I'll show them' attitude." (Llorens/Peters oral history, April 25–26, 2003, lines 308–312).

39. Remembering the early 1950s, Llorens stated: "In those days Western Michigan University had about 4,500 students in total, and about 50 black students. There were no black sororities, so I helped bring Delta Sigma Theta to Western Michigan." (Llorens/Peters oral history, April 25–26, 2003, lines 5043–5045; 3071–3975).

40. Joseph Llorens, PhD, is a scholar and an accomplished artist and educator. He has taught at the elementary through university level, with an emphasis on African American history, culture, and art. Many of Dr. Llorens' paintings are in the Llorens home, and have been exhibited throughout the country.

41. Mosey (1981) identified that science grew out of philosophical inquiry.

42. Mosey (1996) described this trial and error process as a traditional epistemological orientation to practice.

43. Llorens refers to the following occupational therapy definition: "Occupational therapy is any activity, mental or physical, prescribed and guided to aid recovery from disease or injury." (McNary, H., 1954). Henrietta McNary wrote about the relationship between occupational therapy to medicine. McNary defined occupational therapy as "any activity, mental or physical, prescribed and guided to aid recovery from disease or injury." (p. 11). The scope of occupational therapy in H. S. Willard and C. S. Spackman, (Eds.) *Principles of Occupational Therapy*, (2nd ed., p. 15) Philadelphia, PA: J. P. Lippincott.

44. Bing reported discarding his notes. Bing's curriculum vitae however places him at Nebraska Psychiatric Institute College of Medicine, University of Nebraska, Omaha as an Associate In Psychiatry from 1960 until 1961.

45. Although not comprehensive, proceeds from the November 15, 1956, Allenberry Inn, Boiling Springs Conference are archived at the AOTF Wilma West Library. Allenberry Conference, Collection NR RG4, Box NR 73, File NR 529 and Collection RG 4, Box 730, File 530. This collection includes discussion about the therapeutic use of self, group techniques, and occupational, recreation, and art therapies. Most notable are the community members in attendance, including: Wilma West, Beatrice Wade, Gail Fidler, Marion Crampton, Elizabeth Ridgway, Naida Ackley, Frieda Behlen, Genevieve (Sister Mirian Joseph) Cummings, Dwyer Dundon, Marie Louise Franciscus, Mary Frances Heermans, Dale Houston, and Fanny Vanderkooi.

46. Spackman (1954) identified the aim of occupational therapy in treatment of physical disabilities as improving joint motion, muscle strength, developing motor skills, work tolerance, and a "wholesome" psychological reaction. She proposed exercise and therapeutic equipment, like the bicycle saw for knee, hip, and back strengthening and increased range of motion. A picture shows an adult male patient at a Veteran's Administration hospital sitting and cutting wood using a pedal powered jigsaw (p. 168).

47. Licht (1952), considered a friend to occupational therapy according to Fidler and Welles, supported occupational therapist's writing and understanding scientific methods.

48. Scientific knowledge stemming from positivism, a philosophic school of thought in the late 19th century, promoted the use of science and technology to improve well-being by testing and standardizing information (Bunge, 1983; Floris Cohen, 1994; Schon, 1983). Believers in a post-positivistic philosophy in the 1960s questioned the doctrines of positivism that stated that science was absolute, reliable, and authoritative (Kuhn, 1970; Laudan, 1990). When scientists began questioning scientific paradigms and

the authority of science, related discussions began about the relevance of scientific knowledge to the development of professions.

49. Historians and sociologists see knowledge development as a component of professional develop- ment. Looking through broader lenses they identify various frames of reference including functionalism, monopolism, and a systems theory viewpoint (Abbott, 1988; Argyris & Schon, 1974; Balogh, 1991; Bledstein, 1978; Etzioni, 1969; Freidson, 1984; Goode, 1969; Haskell, 1984; Hollinger, 1997, 1965; Larson, 1984; Simpson & Simpson, 1969; Walters, 1997; Wilensky & Lebeau, 1965). Supporters of functionalism examine the structure of organizations, linking form to function to better understand its purpose (Argyris & Schon, 1974; Cantor & Schneider, 1967; Freidson, 1984). Going unchallenged until the 1960s, function- alists believed professionals have the right to decide the nature of their work, and the content of its knowl- edge base (Freidson, 1984; Wilensky & Lebeau, 1965). Functionalism can be challenged for placing too much importance on intellectual elitism, and focusing solely on a profession's internal structure, rather than external interactions with other professions or society. (Bunge, 1983; Floris Cohen, 1994; Schon, 1983).

50. Monopolists state that professions develop knowledge for reasons of power, dominance, and authority (Larson, 1984). Monopolism, similar to functionalism, is limited, appearing to analyze professions in isolation. This seems particularly curious when speaking about political engagements and jurisdictional wars with others. A functionalist and monopolist hybrid exists since the 1970s, viewing expert knowledge as a commodity in the marketplace for power and status, with the most viable profes- sions maintaining an intellectual "elite" and business plan savvy (Brint, 1994).

51. Systems theory describes how professions form through interdependent histories and by sustain- ing jurisdiction (Abbott, 1988). This was evident during Cold War America, when nuclear scientists set off a chain reaction using expert scientific knowledge as a bartering tool that linked scientists with health care, universities, and national policy makers (Balogh, 1991; Walters, 1997).

52. Those involved were Carolyn Baum, Chairperson, Commission on Standards and Ethics; Paul Ellsworth, Chairperson, Commission on Practice; James Garibaldi, Executive Director, AOTA; Kay Grant, Member, Commission on Education; Carole Hays, Vice Speaker, Representative Assembly; Dottie Marsh, Director, Practice Division, AOTA; Nancy Prendergast, Chairperson, Commission on Education; Phil Shannon, Member, Commission on Practice; and Mary Young, Education Division, AOTA.

53. The meeting agenda shows this title. (Bing, 1982, private papers).

54. The branch of the State University of New York was not specified in the agenda documents.

55. Mae Hightower Van Damn was AOTA president when the Representative Assembly Resolution C (1979) passed.

56. "Phil Shannon had tried to become president, running against Mae Hightower. Phil was in the service at the time and he goofed by not getting official permission from his army superiors. When they found out he was a candidate they told him that if he won he would have to resign. If he lost, it would be recorded on his record. He lost, it was smack dab in the middle of the feminist movement." (Bing/Peters oral history, March 7, 2003, lines 1170–1176).

57. Fidler recalled this workshop: "I got a grant to do something about OT education and theory. Educators spent an all-expense-paid week in New York looking at what they taught, and why. It was terrible. They were to come back a second week, but they never did. Theory was a foreign language." (Fidler/Peters oral history, March 6–7, 2003, lines 4122–4199).

58. Grady, Representative Assembly Speaker in 1979 during Hightower–Van Damm's presidency, and close Gilfoyle colleague, would go on to receive the Eleanor Clarke Slagle lectureship and be elected the AOTA presidency after this1983 Scottsdale meeting. In 1983, occupational therapist Fred Sammons, a known AOTA and AOTF financial sponsor, was the creator and senior officer of Fred Sammons, Inc., an adaptive equipment company currently named Sammons Preston Rolyan.

59. Shannon (1977) argued that occupational therapy's "symbiosis" with the medical model and the rehabilitation movement acted as a derailment away from an occupational therapy behavior paradigm, and founding values expressed by Meyers and Slagle. Similarly, Shannon (1993) wrote "philosophical con- sideration for the practice of occupational therapy," chapter 3, pp. 35–42 in S. E. Ryan (Ed.) *The certified occupational therapy assistant*, 2nd ed. Thorofare, New Jersey: Slack.

60. Carolyn Baum is the current AOTA President in 2005. Bing explained a community connection between Jerry Johnson and Carolyn Baum: "Baum really did not 'appear' until the mid to late '70 s, and it was mainly in AOTA. She aligned herself with Jerry Johnson who was president during that time." (Bing/ Peters oral history, February 23, 2003, lines 693–695). Baum worked under Johnson when Johnson was the occupational therapy program director at Washington University in St. Louis, Missouri, 1976 until 1982.

61. Kuhn (1970) challenged the traditional view of an objective science.

62. Kathlyn L. Reed, PhD, OTR, FAOTA was the 1986 Eleanor Clarke Slagle Lecturer and close colleague of community outsider Robert K. Bing. Reed (1986) presented: "Tools of practice: Heritage or baggage?" a philosophical and historical discussion about occupational therapy media in which she recommended that occupational therapy analysis should be based on values and philosophical heritage.

63. The rehabilitation movement grew from a need. Injured and mentally exhausted World War II soldiers returned to their homes, needing occupational therapy services to aid their work force re-entry (Gritzer & Arluke, 1985; Mosey, 1971). President Franklin D. Roosevelt (FDR) understood firsthand rehabilitation efforts, having survived poliomyelitis in 1921. Shifting funds from the Federal Emergency Relief Administration, FDR and his right hand man Harry Hopkins appropriated $70,000 monthly in 1934 and 1935 to provide vocational rehabilitation services to public assistance cases, giving financial sustenance to the movement (Dean, 1972). Vocational rehabilitation grew secondary to New Deal Programs viewing employment as an ultimate goal for all. First Lady Eleanor Roosevelt began health care advocacy work that linked her to occupational therapy leader Eleanor Clarke Slagle.

64. Shannon (1977) saw occupational therapists' involvement in the rehabilitation movement counter-productive and a "derailment" from the profession's humanistic philosophical base.

65. Yerxa spoke about her dismay that Rancho Los Amigos, a renowned rehabilitation center known for its innovative work with polio patients 50 years ago, was closing because of budget deficits. Susan Fox, of the *Los Angeles Times* reported that a federal judge issued a temporary restraining order April 29, 2003, to prevent Los Angeles County from closing the hospital, a controversial issue in California (Fox, April 30, 2003, *Los Angeles Times*).

66. The Flexner Report (1910/1960), funded by the non-profit Carnegie Foundation for the Advancement of Teaching, ensured medicine's authority by limiting the number of qualified medical schools producing physicians. A landmark work in medical history, Flexner's strategy to protect society from less qualified or "under-educated poorly trained physicians" worked positively for doctors. Limiting doctors in the marketplace created a smaller pool deemed the most qualified or professional elite. Medicine, "the men of science," and prestigious educational and medical institutions, such as Harvard and Johns Hopkins, thrived in the public eye, creating a sense of authority (Hall, 1984).

67. Female physicians had a different path in medicine than men, paradoxically excluded in a male-dominated profession, but also aided by the woman's movement. Women physicians positioned themselves in the unwanted (by men) aspects of medicine like public heath, and obstetrics and pediatrics, out of choice and necessity. In contrast, male physicians did not easily relinquish coveted "scientific" practice areas like neurology, surgery, internal medicine, cardiology, or orthopedics to female doctors. Although female physicians were willing to join male ranks as scientists, women were not accepted and continued to make little headway in scientific precincts until the 1960s. With a move away from gender stereotyping, women physicians hoped that the practice of medicine could include nurturance and objective science (Morantz–Sanchez, 1985).

68. Bing, Cromwell, and Wiemer's analyses about physical medicine and physical therapy relations and actions reflect their opinions as occupational therapists. A question beyond the scope of this study is how physical therapy leaders perceived the shift to state licensing and relinquishing the RPT: was this battle won or lost?

69. In 1975 Congress passed Public Law 94-142 (Education of All Handicapped Children Act) now codified as IDEA (Individual with Disabilities Education Act). To receive federal funds, states must develop and implement policies that assure a free appropriate public education to all children with disabilities. Retrieved June 19, 2005 from http://www.scn.org/bk269/94-142.html.

70. Except during World War II, which tended to erase gender discrimination, women scientists remained separate, invisible, or an embarrassment to male dominated science (May, 1988; Rossiter, 1995). Married female scientists worked marginalized jobs. Doctorally educated women held positions as teaching assistants or part-time research assistants in academic settings, particularly if their husbands held full faculty positions at the same institutions. Some institutions did not allow dual appointments, and deferred to male hires. Such discrimination, not uncommon, led to affirmative action policies and legislation.

71. Nationally, new opportunities evolved for women, seen in the Commission on the Status of Women in 1960 under Eleanor Roosevelt, and the 1963 Equal Pay Act legislating equal pay for equal work. Title VII of the Civil Rights Act in 1964 made sexual discrimination in the work place illegal (Solomon, 1985). Leaders of the National Organization of Women (NOW), promoting gender equality, admonished discrimination against women in "professions, science and medicine" (National Organization of Women, 1966). They believed women no longer had to choose between motherhood and career. NOW, characterized as an exclusively white, middle class club of educated women, is criticized for not meeting the needs

of racially diverse, non-college-educated or lower class women (Degler, 1980). Cautiously, feminists in the 1970s continued carving out women's movement gains initiated in the 1960s (Friedan, 1963, 1976; Steinem, 1994; Tobias, 1997). Completing a pendulum swing, a political regrouping occurred leading to a return to an ideological conservatism for women in the 1980s (Faludi, 1991).

72. Nurses struggled for a balance between duty and advancement as scientists. The scientists were considered nursing elite, primarily academics and scholars who were removed from the overwhelming demands of day-to-day practice. Nurses working in male-dominated medical environments continually felt practice demands. Practitioners, generally undervalued for their scientific or professional training, compliantly knuckled under to physician demands, having little autonomy. Nursing's nurturant and caring values were criticized for causing image problems and allowed it to be labeled as a lower status or semi-profession (Etzioni, 1969). Nursing's jurisdictional conflicts for autonomy are similar to, but different from, occupational therapy's. Nurses came from a split class system in the 1850s, the untrained immigrant and older house domestics from the lower working class, and the educated middle and upper-middle class educated women who linked service and science (Reverby, 1987). Occupational therapy in the 1920s was thought to be a more homogeneous cohort of upper-middle class women that remained small in numbers compared to the larger, more established, nursing profession. The similarities lie in both female professions' quest for a unique (from medicine) science-based body of knowledge. The connection between nursing and occupational therapy goes beyond their quest to separate from medicine. Nursing played an important role in occupational therapy's founding, which established a tradition that carried into the post World War II years.

73. Different from popular belief, women's role conflicts at home did not improve with technological advances. For example, women using household technology such as washing machines and vacuum cleaners did not gain leisure time, rather additional hours to work outside the home (Cowan, 1983).

74. Wiemer explained: "In private, Slagle's colleagues called her Suzy Slagle" (Wiemer lines 1317–1322). Other therapists who emulated Slagle's humanitarianism, white upper-middle class value system, and accomplishments, were called the Suzy Slagles.

REFERENCES

Abbott, A. (1988). *The system of professions: An essay on division of expert labor.* Chicago, IL: University of Chicago Press.

Abreu, B. C., Peloquin, S. M., & Ottenbacher, K. (1998). Competence in scientific inquiry and research. *American Journal of Occupational Therapy, 52,* 751–759.

Adams, S. H. (1984). *Life of Henry Forster, M.D., founder Clifton Springs sanitarium.* Reprinted for Clifton Springs library. Canandaigua, NY: Humphrey Press.

American Occupational Therapy Association and American Occupational Therapy Foundation. (2004). Research priorities and the parameters of practice for occupational therapy: Established 1999; Reaffirmed 2003 by AOTA and AOTF. *OT Practice, 9*(4), 20–21. Bethesda, MD: Author.

American Occupational Therapy Association. (1967). *Then 1917 and now 1967: 50th anniversary American occupational therapy association.* New York, NY: Author.

American Occupational Therapy Association. (1969). American occupational therapy association bestows award of merit on Ruth Brunyate and Myra McDaniel. *American Journal of Occupational Therapy, XXIII,* 113. New York, NY: Author.

American Occupational Therapy Association. (1975). Honorary awards presented at the 1974 annual AOTA conference: Fiorentino and Cromwell. *American Journal of Occupational Therapy, 29*(1), 8–9. Rockville, MD: Author.

American Occupational Therapy Association. (1978). Research institute at conference: Joint foundation and specialty sections enterprise features Yerxa, Ayres, West and Llorens. *OT Newspaper, 32*(1), 7. Rockville, MD: Author.

American Occupational Therapy Association. (1979, January). Resolutions. *Occupational Therapy Newspaper, 33*, 5.

American Occupational Therapy Association. (1981). Honorary doctor of science degree conferred on Ellie Gilfoyle. *Occupational Therapy Newspaper, 35*(7), 1. Rockville, MD: Author.

American Occupational Therapy Association. (1984, January). President Bing visits White House for signing of proclamation for decade of disabled persons. *Occupational Therapy Newspaper, 38*(1), 1–10.

American Occupational Therapy Association. (1986). Meet Ellie Gilfoyle: Profile of AOTA's new president. *Occupational Therapy News, 40*(5), 1, 20. Rockville, MD: Author.

American Occupational Therapy Association. (1988). Gilfoyle named associate dean at Colorado state university. *Occupational Therapy News, 42*(9), 1, 19. Rockville, MD: Author.

American Occupational Therapy Association. (1998a). Honoring a lifetime of service: Ruth Brunyate Wiemer becomes the fifth recipient of the Wilma L. West AOTA-AOTF president's commendation. *OT Week*, April 16, 1998, p. 11. Bethesda, MD: Author.

American Occupational Therapy Association. (1998b). Special honors for special people: Florence Stattel, award of merit. *OT Week*, April 16, 1998, p. 12. Bethesda, MD: Author.

American Occupational Therapy Association. (2001a). AOTA 2000 member compensation survey. *OT Practice, 6*(9), 20. Bethesda, MD: Author.

American Occupational Therapy Association. (2001b). Streamline policy development and decision making processes. Strategic Plan Ad Hoc Group Report, R. Jones, Chairperson. Bethesda, MD: Author.

American Occupational Therapy Foundation. (1975). The first decade: 1965–1975. *American Journal of Occupational Therapy, 29*, 636–640.

American Occupational Therapy Foundation. (1982). The 1981 certificate of appreciation: Llorens and Crampton. *American Journal of Occupational Therapy, 36*, 195.

American Occupational Therapy Foundation. (1983). Academy of research award presentations: Ayres, Reilly, Yerxa. *American Journal of Occupational Therapy, 37*, 631–632.

American Occupational Therapy Foundation. (1998). Carlotta Welles: A treasure of our profession. *AOTF Connection, 6*(3), 1, 4.

American Occupational Therapy Foundation. (2000a). AOTF mission statement. *AOTF Connection, 8*, 3.

American Occupational Therapy Foundation. (2000b). A twenty-year history of research funding in occupational therapy. *American Journal of Occupational Therapy, 54*, 441–442.

American Occupational Therapy Foundation. (2002a). Occupational therapy honors Gail Fidler. *AOTF Connection, 9*(2), 4.

American Occupational Therapy Foundation. (2002b). Foundation mourns loss of friend—Florence Stattel. *AOTF Connection, 9*(2), 6.

American Occupational Therapy Foundation. (2002c, Summer). Gail Fidler honored. *AOTF Connection, 9*.

Appleby, J., Hunt, L., & Jacob, M. (1994). *Telling the truth about history*. New York, NY: Norton.

Argyris, C., & Schon, D. A. (1974). *Theory in practice: Increasing professional effectiveness*. San Francisco, CA: Jossey–Bass.

Aristotle (1980). *The nicomachean ethics*. (D. Ross, Trans.; J. L. Ackrill & J. O. Urmon. Revision). New York, NY: Oxford University Press. (Original work published 1925).

Ayres, A. J. (1955a). Proprioceptive facilitation through upper extremities; Part I: Background. *American Journal of Occupational Therapy, IX*, 1–9.

Ayres, A. J. (1955b). Proprioceptive facilitation elicited through upper extremities; Part II: Application. *American Journal of Occupational Therapy, IX*, 57–58, 76.

Ayres, A. J. (1955c). Proprioceptive facilitation elicited through upper extremities; Part III. *American Journal of Occupational Therapy, IX*, 121–126, 143.

Ayres, A. J. (1963). The development of perceptual-motor abilities: A theoretical basis for treatment of dysfunction. *American Journal of Occupational Therapy, XVII*, 221–225.

Ayres, A. J. (1972). *Sensory integration and learning disorders*. Los Angeles, CA: Western Psychological.

Ayres, A. J. (1976). The effect of sensory integrative therapy on learning disabled children. Unpublished final report of a research project supported by the Center for the Study of Sensory Integrative Dysfunction and the Valentine-Kline Foundation 1974–1975–1976. Los Angeles, CA: University of Southern California.

Ayres, A. J. (1979). *Sensory integration and the child*. Los Angeles, CA: Western Psychological.

Balogh, B. (1991). *Chain reaction: Expert debate and public participation in American commercial and nuclear power, 1945–1975*. New York, NY: Cambridge University Press.

Barris, R., Kielhofner, G., & Watts, J. H. (1988). *Bodies of knowledge in psychosocial practice*. Thorofare, NJ: Slack.

Barzun, J., & Graff, H. F. (1970). *The modern researcher*. New York, NY: Harcourt Brace.

Bennis, W. (1989). *Why leaders can't lead*. San Francisco, CA: Josey–Bass.

Berg, J. (1997). Laying the groundwork for modern practice. *OT Week, 11*(16), 14–16.

Bing, R. K. (1954, January). Parent–child relations with respect to the handicapped child. Unpublished paper, the Institute for Child Study, University of Maryland, College Park, MD.

Bing, R. K. (1958, May). He can pitch, can't he? Paper presented for The Crippled Child seminar, National Society for Crippled Children and Adults, location unknown.

Bing, R. K. (1961). Methods of research for the occupational therapist: A handbook. Paper presented to Illinois State Psychiatric Institute, Chicago, IL.

Bing, R. K. (1962, June). Department of occupational therapy: A proposed program. Paper presented to Moosehaven department of occupational therapy, Orange Park, FL.

Bing, R. K. (1969a, December 31). Requisites for relevance: Changing concepts in occupational therapy education. *Annals of the New York Academy of Sciences, 166*(3), 1020–1026.

Bing, R. K. (1969b). Methods of measurement and evaluation in psychiatric dysfunction. In L. J. Zamir (Ed.), *Expanding dimensions in rehabilitation: A reference for the health professional* (pp. 131–195). Springfield, IL: Thomas.

Bing, R. K. (1981). Occupational therapy revisited: A parphrastic journey. *American Journal of Occupational Therapy, 35*, 499–518.

Bing, R. K. (1982, July 12). Handwritten notes of R. K. Bing, who was attending The Philosophical Base Project of Occupational Therapy: Phase 3, Slagle Meeting, July 12–16, 1982, Phoenix, AZ (Bing private collection).

Bing, R. K. (1983a). Beliefs at a new beginning. *American Journal of Occupational Therapy, 37*, 375–379.

Bing, R. K. (1983b). The industry, the art, the philosophy of history. *American Journal of Occupational Therapy, 37*, 800–801.

Bing, R. K. (1984a). Living forward, understanding backward: Part I. *American Journal of Occupational Therapy, 38*, 363–366.

Bing, R. K. (1984b). Living forward, understanding backward: Part II. *American Journal of Occupational Therapy, 38*, 435–439.

Bing, R. K. (1984c). To survive, to become: Our way of life. *American Journal of Occupational Therapy, 38*, 785–790.

Bing, R. K. (1987). Who originated the term "occupational therapy"? Letter to the editor. *American Journal of Occupational Therapy, 41*, 3.

Bing, R. K. (1993). Living forward, understanding backward: A history of occupational therapy principles. In S. E. Ryan (Ed.), *The certified occupational therapy assistant: Principles, concepts and techniques* (2nd ed., pp. 3–20). Thorofare, NJ: Slack.

Bing, R. K. (1995). Forward. In V. Quiroga (Ed.), *Occupational therapy: The first 30 years 1900–1930* (pp. 3–10). Bethesda, MD: American Occupational Therapy Association.

Bing, R. K. (1997). "And teach agony to sing": An afternoon with Eleanor Clarke Slagle. *American Journal of Occupational Therapy, 51*, 220–227.

Bledstein, B. J. (1978). *The culture of professionalism: The middle class and the development of higher education in America.* New York, NY: Norton.

Bloch, M. (1953). *The historian's craft.* New York, NY: Vintage Books.

Bloom, B. L. (1977). *Community mental health: A general introduction.* Belmont, CA: Wadsworth.

Boston School of Occupational Therapy: Making history from the outset. (2004, Winter). *Copy Editor, 4, 2.*

Bowman, I. A., & Sherer, B. E. (n.d.). *Guide to the archives of the American Occupational Therapy Association.* The Truman G. Blocker, Jr., History of Medicine Collections, Moody Medical Library, The University of Texas Medical Branch, Galveston, TX.

Bowman, O. J. (1989). A. Jean Ayres 1920–1988: Therapist, scholar, scientist and teacher. *American Journal of Occupational Therapy, 43*, 479–480.

Brandt, A. M. (1997). "Just say no": Risk, behavior and disease in twentieth-century America. In R. G. Walters (Ed.), *Scientific authority and twentieth-century America* (pp. 82–98). Baltimore, MD: Johns Hopkins University Press.

Brint, S. (1994). *In an age of experts: The changing role of professionals in politics and public life.* Princeton, NJ: Princeton University Press.

Brooks, P. C. (1969). *Research in archives: The use of unpublished primary sources.* Chicago, IL: Chicago University Press.

Brown, J. (1997). Crime, commerce and contagionism: The political language of public health and popularization of germ theory in the United States, 1870–1950. In R. G. Walters (Ed.), *Scientific authority in twentieth-century America* (pp. 53–81). Baltimore, MD: Johns Hopkins University Press.

Brunyate, R. W. (1954a). Occupational therapy for patients with cerebral palsy. In H. S. Willard & C. S. Spackman (Eds.) *Principles of occupational therapy*, (2nd ed., pp. 301–329). Philadelphia, PA: Lippincott.

Brunyate, R. W. (1954b). A study of the use of magnetic toys in the treatment of cerebral palsied children. *American Journal of Occupational Therapy, VIII*, 151–155.

Brunyate, R. W. (1958). Powerful levers in little common things. *American Journal of Occupational Therapy, XII*, 4, part II, 193–202.

Brunyate, R. W. (1962). Graphs, their value as a record form in the management of cerebral palsy. *American Journal of Occupational Therapy, XVI*, 13–21.

Brunyate, R. W. (1963a). The student in pre-clinical education: Impressions of a clinically oriented therapist. *American Journal of Occupational Therapy, XVIII*, 181–186.

Brunyate, R. W. (1963b). Occupational therapy for patients with cerebral palsy. In H. S. Willard, & C. S. Spackman (Eds.), *Occupational therapy*, (3rd ed., pp. 264–307).

Brunyate, R. W. (1964). From the president: Graduate education. *American Journal of Occupational Therapy, XVIII*, 68–69.

Brunyate, R. W. (1966). Keynote address 45th annual conference Miami, Florida. *American Journal of Occupational Therapy, XX*, 9–16.

Brunyate, R. W. (1967a). From the president: A modification of role for nursing home service. *American Journal of Occupational Therapy, XXI*(3), 126–127.

Brunyate, R. W. (1967b). After fifty years, what stature do we hold? *American Journal of Occupational Therapy, XXI*, 262–267.

Brunyate, R. W. (1968). *Maryland state department of health: Guidelines for establishing services and recommended standards for occupational therapy and activity programs.* Baltimore, MD: Maryland State Department of Health.

Brunyate, R. W. (1970). Nationally speaking: Medicare, public law 80–97. *American Journal of Occupational Therapy, XXIV*, 89–90.

Brunyate, R. W., & Phelps, W. M. (1950). Occupational therapy in the treatment of cerebral palsy. In W. R. Dunton, & S. Licht (Eds.), *Occupational therapy: Principles and practice* (pp. 173–187). Springfield, IL: Thomas.

Bunge, M. (1983). *Epistemology and methodology I: Treatise on basic philosophy.* Dordrecht, Holland: D. Reidel Publishing.

Burke, J. P. (1996). Moving occupation into treatment: Clinical interpretation of "legitimizing occupational therapy's knowledge." *American Journal of Occupational Therapy, 50*, 635–638.

Burke, J. P., & De Poy, E. (1991). An emerging view of mastery, excellence and leadership in occupational therapy practice. *American Journal of Occupational Therapy, 45*, 1027–1032.

Cantor, N. F., & Schneider, R. I. (1967). *How to study history*. Wheeling, IL: Harlan Davis.

Cayleff, S. E. (1987). *Wash and be healed: The water-cure movement and women's health*. Philadelphia, PA: Temple University Press.

Christiansen, C. H. (1981). Toward resolution of crisis: Research requisites in occupational therapy. *Occupational Therapy Journal of Research, 1*(2), 115–124.

Clark, F., Zemke, R., Frank, G., Parham, D., Neville–Jan, A., Hendricks, C., ... Abreu, B. (1993). Dangers inherent in the partition of occupational therapy and occupational science. *American Journal of Occupational Therapy, 47*, 184–186.

Clark, F. A., Parham, D., Carlson, M. E., Frank, G., Jackson, J., Pierce, D., ... Zemke, R. (1991). Occupational science: Academic innovation in the service of occupational therapy's future. *American Journal of Occupational Therapy, 45*, 300–310.

Clark, P. N. (1979). Human development through occupation: A philosophy and conceptual model for practice, part 2. *American Journal of Occupational Therapy, 33*, 577–585.

Clarke, L. (1989). New ideas on the division of labor. [Review of the book *The system of professions*.]. *Sociological Forum, 4*(2), 281–289.

Cohen, D. W. (1994). *The combing of history*. Chicago, IL: University of Chicago Press.

Colman, W. (1984). A study of educational policy setting in occupational therapy 1918–1981. Doctoral dissertation, New York University, New York, NY.

Colman, W. (1992). Maintaining autonomy: The struggles between occupational therapy and physical medicine. *American Journal of Occupational Therapy, 46*, 63–70.

Coontz, S. (2000). *The way we never were: American families and the nostalgia trap*. New York, NY: Basic Books. (Original work published 1992).

Cowan, R. S. (1983). *More work for mother: The ironies of household technology from the open hearth to the microwave*. New York, NY: Basic Books.

Cox, R. C., & West, W. L. (1982). *Fundamentals of research for health professionals*. Rockville, MD: American Occupational Therapy Foundation & Ramsco.

Crampton, M. W. (1946). Musical magic. *Occupational Therapy and Rehabilitation, 25*, 207–208.

Crampton, M. W. (1950). Group therapy. *Massachusetts Association for Occupational Therapy Newsletter, 24*(4), 1–2.

Crampton, M. W. (1961). Occupational therapy assistants: Trends and development in certification. Proceedings of American Occupational Therapy 1961 conference, Detroit, MI, (pp. 79–86).

Crampton, M. W. (1967a). Nationally speaking: Council on development. *American Journal of Occupational Therapy, XXI*, 54–55.

Crampton, M. W. (1967b). Educational upheaval, occupational therapy assistants. *American Journal of Occupational Therapy, XXI*, 317–320.

Crampton, M. W. (1969). Project report: Development of teaching materials for occupational therapy assistants. Number 543-T-69, Rehabilitation Services Administration, Department of Health Education and Welfare, Boston, MA: Medical Foundation.

Crampton, M. W., & Anderegg, G. F. (1961). Educational weaknesses and occupational stress: A survey. *American Journal of Occupational Therapy, XV,*
233–241, 270.

Crampton, M. W., & MacDonald, J. C. (1973). Report on foundation's relationship to
association's task force on social issues. *American Journal of Occupational
Therapy, 27,* 115–116.

Cromwell, F. S. (1959). A procedure for pre-vocational evaluation. *American Journal
of Occupational Therapy, XIII,* 1–4.

Cromwell, F. S. (1968a). Know your delegates. *American Journal of Occupational
Therapy, XXII,* 4–7.

Cromwell, F. S. (1968b). The executive board. *American Journal of Occupational
Therapy, XXII,* 60–65.

Cromwell, F. S. (1968c). Meet your headquarters. *American Journal of Occupational
Therapy, XXII,* 155–159.

Cromwell, F. S. (1968d). The affiliate association. *American Journal of Occupational
Therapy, XXII,* 255–257.

Cromwell, F. S. (1968e). The newest of our member catergories: the COTA. *American
Journal of Occupational Therapy, XXII,* 377–382.

Cromwell, F. S. (1969a). Nationally speaking: Highlights of our annual meeting in
Portland. *American Journal of Occupational Therapy, XXIII,* 5–7.

Cromwell, F. S. (1969b). Nationally speaking: The occupational therapist's
thoughts on changes and innovations in education and health care for the
allied health professions. *American Journal of Occupational Therapy, XXIII,*
109–112.

Cromwell, F. S. (1969c). Nationally speaking: Change and a commitment to action.
American Journal of Occupational Therapy, XXIII, 297.

Cromwell, F. S. (1969d). Nationally speaking: The here and now demands of
practice. *American Journal of Occupational Therapy, XXIII,* 381–385.

Cromwell, F. S. (1969e). Nationally speaking: AOTA budget. *American Journal of
Occupational Therapy, XXIII,* 469–471.

Cromwell, F. S. (1970a). Growth and restraint potentials in occupational therapy
education. *American Journal of Occupational Therapy, XXIV,* 253–254.

Cromwell, F. S. (1970b). Nationally speaking: Issues affecting the profession.
American Journal of Occupational Therapy, XXIV, 471–472.

Cromwell, F. S. (1970c). Factors affecting personnel utilization. *American Journal of
Occupational Therapy, XXIV,* 541–542.

Cromwell, F. S. (1972a). Nationally speaking: Standards for accreditation of
hospitals. *American Journal of Occupational Therapy, 26,* 3A.

Cromwell, F. S. (1972b). Nationally speaking: Joint commission on accreditation of
hospitals. *American Journal of Occupational Therapy, 26,* 3A.

Cromwell, F. S. (1972c). Statement to the Joint Commission on Accreditation of
Hospitals, Chicago, Illinois. *American Journal of Occupational Therapy, 26,*
3A–5A.

Cromwell, F. S. (1972d). Nationally speaking: National office relocation. *American
Journal of Occupational Therapy, 26,* 3A.

Cromwell, F. S. (1973a). Nationally speaking: 1973 renewal. *American Journal of
Occupational Therapy, 27,* 3A.

Cromwell, F. S. (1973b). Qua Vadis: American Medical Association/American Occupational Therapy Association. *American Journal of Occupational Therapy, 27,* 7A–9A.

Cromwell, F. S. (1973c). Professional self-evaluation tool. *American Journal of Occupational Therapy, 27,* 5A–12A.

Cromwell, F. S. (1973d). Accreditation, certification, licensure, registration. *American Journal of Occupational Therapy, 27,* 307–308.

Cromwell, F. S. (1973e). Nationally speaking: Concluding six years of sharing. *American Journal of Occupational Therapy, 27,* 451–452.

Cromwell, F. S. (1977). Eleanor Clarke Slagle: The leader, the woman. *American Journal of Occupational Therapy, 31,* 645–648.

Cromwell, F. S. (1979a). Know and use current federal legislation. *American Journal of Occupational Therapy, 33,* 9–10.

Cromwell, F. S. (1979b). External influences impacting occupational therapy. In *Occupational Therapy: 2001,* papers presented at the special session of the representative assembly, November 8–12, 1978, in Scottsdale, AZ, (pp. 37–41). Rockville, MD: American Occupational Therapy Association.

Cromwell, F. S. (1985). Work-related programming in occupational therapy: Its roots, course and prognosis. In F. S. Cromwell (Ed.), *Work-Related Programs in Occupational Therapy* (pp. 9–25). New York, NY: Haworth Press.

Cromwell, F. S., & Kielhofner, G. W. (1976). An educational strategy for occupational therapy community service. *American Journal of Occupational Therapy, 30*(10), 629–633.

Custard, C. (1998). Tracing research methodology in occupational therapy. *American Journal of Occupational Therapy, 52,* 676–683.

Dean, R. J. (1972). *New life for millions: Rehabilitation for America's disabled.* New York, NY: Hastings House.

Degler, C. N. (1980). *At odds: Women and the American family in America from the revolution to the present.* New York, NY: Oxford University Press.

Dickson, D. (1988). *The new politics of science.* Chicago, IL: University of Chicago Press.

Di Maggio, P. (1989). Book review. [Review of the book *The system of professions*]. *American Journal of Sociology, 95*(2), 534–535.

Duchek, J. M., & Thessing, V. (1996). Is the use of life history and narrative in clinical practice fundable research? *American Journal of Occupational Therapy, 50,* 393–395.

Dunton, W. R. (1947). History and development of occupational therapy. In H. S. Willard, & C. S. Spackman (Eds.), *Principles of occupational therapy* (pp. 1–9). Philadelphia, PA: Lippincott.

Dunton, W. R. (1950). History of occupational therapy. In W. R. Dunton & S. Licht (Eds) *Occupational therapy: Principles and practice* (pp. 3–7). Springfield, IL: Thomas.

Dunton, W. R., & Licht, S. (1950). *Occupational therapy principles and practice.* Springfield, IL: Charles C. Thomas.

Elgin, C. (1998). Epistemology's end. In L. M. Alcoff (Ed.), *Epistemology the big question* (pp. 26–40). Malden, MA: Blackwell.

Engleke Holdeman, E. (1954). Occupational therapy for patients with anterior polio-myelitis. In H. S. Willard and C. S. Spackman (Eds.), *Principles of occupational therapy* (2nd ed., pp. 256–267). Philadelphia, PA: Lippincott.

Etzioni, A. (Ed.) (1969). *The semi-professions and their organization: Teachers, nurses, social workers*. New York, NY: Free Press.

Faeser, E. (1949). Meeting of the house of delegates American Occupational Therapy Association, board of management minutes: New business. *American Journal of Occupational Therapy, IV*, 132.

Faludi, S. (1991). *Backlash: The undeclared war against American women*. New York, NY: Anchor Books.

Fidler, G., & Velde, B. (1999). *Activities: Reality and symbol*. Thorofare, NJ: Slack.

Fidler, G. S. (1957). The role of occupational therapy in a multi-discipline approach to psychiatric illness. *American Journal of Occupational Therapy, XI*(1), 8–12, 35.

Fidler, G. S. (1958). Some unique contributions of occupational therapy in treatment of the schizophrenic. *American Journal of Occupational Therapy, XII*, 9–12, 36.

Fidler, G. S. (1964). Guide to planning and measuring growth experiences in the clinical affiliation. *American Journal of Occupational Therapy, XVIII*, 240–243.

Fidler, G. S. (1966a). Learning as a growth process: A conceptual framework for professional education. *American Journal of Occupational Therapy, XX*, 1–8.

Fidler, G. S. (1966b). A second look at work as a primary force in rehabilitation and treatment. *American Journal of Occupational Therapy, XX*, 72–74.

Fidler, G. S. (1969). The task-oriented group as a context for treatment. *American Journal of Occupational Therapy, XXIII*, 43–48.

Fidler, G. S. (1977). From plea to mandate. *American Journal of Occupational Therapy, 31*, 653–655.

Fidler, G. S. (1979a). Professional or non professional. In Occupational therapy: 2001, papers presented at the special session of the representative assembly, November 8–12, 1978, in Scottsdale, AZ (pp. 31–36). Rockville, MD: American Occupational Therapy Association.

Fidler, G. S. (1979b). Specialization: Implications for education. *American Journal of Occupational Therapy, 33*, 34–35.

Fidler, G. S. (1981). From crafts to competence. *American Journal of Occupational Therapy, 35*, 567–573.

Fidler, G. S. (1982). The lifestyle performance profile: An organizing frame. In B. Hemphill (Ed.), *The evaluative process in psychiatric occupational therapy* (pp. 43–47). Thorofare, NJ: Slack.

Fidler, G. S. (1983). Overview of occupational therapy in mental health. White paper prepared by the American Occupational Therapy Association Task Group of the American Psychiatric Association (APA) Psychiatric Therapies, G. S. Fidler, chair, submitted May 1981. Approved by the Executive Board of the American Occupation Therapy Association, July 1981. Rockville: MD.

Fidler, G. S. (1984). *Design of rehabilitation service in psychiatric hospital settings*. Laurel, MD: Ramsco.

Fidler, G. S. (1988). The life-style performance profile. In S. C. Robertson (Ed.), *Mental health focus: Skills for assessment and treatment* (section 3, pp. 35–40). Rockville, MD: American Occupational Therapy Association.

Fidler, G. S. (1994). The psychosocial core of occupational therapy: Position paper. Prepared for the Commission on Practice, American Occupational

Therapy Association. Rockville, MD: American Occupational Therapy Association.

Fidler, G. S. (1997). Forward. In C. Christiansen & C. Baum (Eds.), *Occupational therapy: Enabling function and well-being*. Thorofare, NJ: Slack.

Fidler, G. S., & Fidler, J. W. (1954). *Introduction to psychiatric occupational therapy*. New York, NY: MacMillan.

Fidler, G. S., & Fidler, J. W. (1963). *Occupational therapy: A communication process in psychiatry*. New York, NY: MacMillan.

Fidler, G. S., & Fidler, J. W. (1978). Doing and becoming: Purposeful action and self-actualization. *American Journal of Occupational Therapy, 32*, 305–310.

Fidler, G. S., & Fidler, J. W. (1983). Doing and becoming: The occupational therapy experience. In G. Kielhofner (Ed.), *Health through occupation: Theory and practice in occupational therapy* (pp. 267–279). Philadelphia, PA: F. A. Davis.

Fiorentino, M. R. (1975). Occupational therapy: Realization to activation. *American Journal of Occupational Therapy, 29*, 15–21.

Fischer, D. H. (1970). *Historians' fallacies: Toward a logic of historical thought*. New York, NY: Harper and Row.

Flexner, A. (1960). *The Flexner report on medical education in the United States and Canada 1910*. Commissioned by the Carnegie Foundation for the Advancement of Teaching. Washington, D.C.: Science and Health Publications. (Original work published 1910).

Floris Cohen, H. (1994). *A scientific revolution: A historiographical inquiry*. Chicago, IL: University of Chicago Press.

Fox, S. (2003, April 30). Judge blocks Rancho's closing. *Los Angeles Times*. Retrieved from http://articles.latimes.com/2003/apr/30/local/me-supes30

Freidan, B. (1963). *The feminine mystique*. New York, NY: Dell.

Freidland, J. (1998). Occupational therapy and rehabilitation: An awkward alliance. *American Journal of Occupational Therapy, 52*, 373–380.

Freidson, E. (1984). Are professions necessary? In T. L. Haskel (Ed.), *The authority of experts: Studies in history and theory* (pp. 3–27). Bloomington, IN: Indiana University Press.

Frisch, M. (1990). *A shared authority: Essays on the craft and meaning of oral and public history*. Albany, NY: State University of New York Press.

Froehlich, J. (1992). Proud and visible as occupational therapists. *American Journal of Occupational Therapy, 46*, 1042–1044.

Fuchs, V. R. (1988). *Women's quest for economic equality*. Cambridge, MA: Harvard University Press.

Gevitz, N. (1988). *Other healers: Unorthodox medicine in America*. Baltimore, MD: Johns Hopkins University Press.

Gifford, F. L. (1984). *The early history of the Village of Clifton Springs. Clifton Springs, New York 125th anniversary of incorporation. A souvenir booklet*. Canandaigua, NY: W. F. Humphrey Press.

Gifford, F. L. (2000). *Clifton Springs hospital and clinic 150th anniversary: 1850–2000*. Clifton Springs, NY: Clifton Springs Historical Society.

Gilfoyle, E., & Hays, C. (1979). Occupational therapy roles and functions in education of school-based handicapped student. *American Journal of Occupational Therapy, 33*, 565–576.

Gilfoyle, E. M. (1984). Transformation of a profession. *American Journal of Occupational Therapy, 38*, 575–584.

Gilfoyle, E. M. (1986a). Taking care of ourselves as health care providers. *American Journal of Occupational Therapy, 40*, 387–389.

Gilfoyle, E. M. (1986b). Professional directions: Management in action. *American Journal of Occupational Therapy, 40*, 593–596.

Gilfoyle, E. M. (1986c). Welcoming remarks. Proceedings of Target Occupational Therapy Education 2000: Promoting Excellence in Education, June 22–26, 1986, Nashville, TN, pp. 3–5. Rockville, MD, American Occupational Therapy Association.

Gilfoyle, E. M. (1987a). Leadership and management. *American Journal of Occupational Therapy, 41*, 281–283.

Gilfoyle, E. M. (1987b). Creative partnerships: The profession's plan. *American Journal of Occupational Therapy, 41*, 779–781.

Gilfoyle, E. M. (1987c). Letter from the president. *Mental Health Special Interest Section Newsletter, 10*(1), 1.

Gilfoyle, E. M. (1988). Partnerships for the future. *American Journal of Occupational Therapy, 42*, 485–488.

Gilfoyle, E. M., & Christiansen, C. H. (1987). Research: The quest for the truth and the key to excellence. *American Journal of Occupational Therapy, 41*, 7–8.

Gilfoyle, E. M., & Grady, A. P. (1971). Cognitive-perceptual-motor behavior. In H. S. Willard & C. S. Spackman (Eds.), *Occupational Therapy*, (4th ed., pp. 401–479). Philadelphia, PA: Lippincott.

Gilfoyle, E. M., & Grady, A. P. (1978). Posture and movement: Theory of spatiotemporal adaptation. In H. L. Hopkins & H. D. Smith (Eds), *Willard and Spackman's Occupational Therapy*, (5th ed., pp. 58–81). Philadelphia, PA: Lippincott.

Gilfoyle, E. M., Grady, A. P., & Moore, J. C. (1981). *Children adapt.* Thorofare, NJ: Slack.

Gillette, N., & Kielhofner, G. (1979). The impact of specialization on the professionalization or the survival of occupational therapy. *American Journal of Occupational Therapy, 33*, 20–29.

Gilligan Kapcar, M. B. (1976). Developmental stages of occupational therapy and the feminist movement. *American Journal of Occupational Therapy, 30*, 560–567.

Goode, W. J. (1969). Theoretical limits of professionalization. In A. Etzioni (Ed.), *Semi professions and their organization: Teachers, nurses, social workers* (pp. 266–313). New York, NY: Free Press.

Gottschalk, L. (1969). *Understanding history: A primer of historical method.* New York, NY: Knopf.

Gritzer, G., & Arluke, A. (1985). *The making of rehabilitation: A political economy of medical specialization, 1890–1980.* Berkeley, CA: University of California Press.

Hall, D. (1984). Social foundations of professional credibility: Linking the medical profession to higher education in Connecticut and Massachusettes 1700–1830. In T. L. Haskel, (Ed.), *The authority of experts: Studies in history and theory* (pp. 107–141). Bloomington, IN: Indiana University Press.

Haskel, T. L. (Ed.) (1984). *The authority of experts: Studies in history and theory.* Bloomington, IN: Indiana University Press.

Hollinger, D. A. (1997). How wide the circle are we? In R. G. Walters (Ed.), *Scientific authority and twentieth-century America* (pp. 13–31). Baltimore, MD: Johns Hopkins University Press.

Hollis, I. L. (1979). The 1979 Eleanor Clarke Slagle lecture: Remember? *American Journal of Occupational Therapy, 33,* 493–499.

Hopkins, H. L. (1978). A historical perspective of occupational therapy. In H. L. Hopkins & H. D. Smith (Eds.), *Willard and Spackman's occupational therapy* (5th ed., pp. 3–23). Philadelphia, PA: Lippincott.

Huss, A. J. (1977). Touch with care or a caring touch? *American Journal of Occupational Therapy, 31,* 11–18.

Jantzen, A. C. (1972a). Some characteristics of female occupational therapists, 1970: Part I. *American Journal of Occupational Therapy, 26,* 19–26.

Jantzen, A. C. (1972b). Some characteristics of female occupational therapists part II: Employment patterns of female occupational therapists, 1970. *American Journal of Occupational Therapy, 26,* 67–77.

Jantzen, A. C., Pershing, R., Bates, E., Booth, M., Burns, C., Hoffman, C., . . . Laurencelle, P. (1964). Graduate degrees held by occupational therapists: March 1963. *American Journal of Occupational Therapy, XVIII,* 152–157.

Joe, B. E. (1998). A pioneer of modern occupational therapy. *OT Week, 12*(18), 14.

Johnson, J. A. (1973). Occupational therapy: A model for the future. *American Journal of Occupational Therapy, 27,* 1–7.

Johnson, J. A. (1978). Issues in education: Report of the ad hoc committee on education. *American Journal of Occupational Therapy, 32,* 355–358.

Johnson, J. A., Crampton, M., Kinnealey, M., MacDonald, J., Rothenberg, S., Schmidt, E., . . . West, W. (1972). Report of the task force on social issues. Submitted March 7, 1972, to the American Occupation Therapy Association, by J. A. Johnson, Chairperson. *American Journal of Occupational Therapy, 26,* 332–359.

Jones, J. L. (1992). Therefore be it resolved: 25 years of delegate/representative assembly legislation. *American Journal of Occupational Therapy, 46,* 72–78.

Kaestle, C. F. (1996). Standards of evidence in historical research. *History of Education Quarterly, 32,* 361–366.

Kahman, W. (1950). Nationally speaking: From the president. *American Journal of Occupational Therapy, IV,* 22–23.

Kahmann, W. C., & West, W. (1947). Occupational therapy in the United States army hospitals: World War II, parts 1 & 2. In H. S. Willard & C. S. Spackman (Eds.), *Principles of occupational therapy* (pp. 329–370). Philadelphia, PA: Lippincott.

Kielhofner, G. (1980). A model of human occupation, part 1: Conceptual framework and content. *American Journal of Occupational Therapy, 34,* 657–663.

Kielhofner, G. (1997). *Conceptual foundations of occupational therapy.* Philadelphia, PA: F. A. Davis.

Kielhofner, G., & Burke, J. P. (1977). Occupational therapy after 60 years: An account of changing identity and knowledge. *American Journal of Occupational Therapy, 31,* 675–689.

Kielhofner, G., & Burke, J. P. (1983). The evolution of knowledge and practice in occupational therapy: Past, present and future. In G. Kielhofner (Ed.), *Health through occupation: Theory and practice in occupational therapy* (pp. 3–10). Philadelphia, PA: Davis.

Kirkpatrick, S. A., & Locke, E. A. (1991). Leadership: Do traits matter? *Academy of Management Executives, 5,* 48–60.

Kuhn, T. (1970). *The structure of scientific revolutions.* Chicago, IL: University of Chicago Press.

Larson, M. S. (1984). The production of expertise and constitution of expert power. In. T. L. Haskell (Ed.), *The authority of experts: Studies in history and theory* (pp. 28–80). Bloomington, IN: Indiana University Press.

Lash, J. P. (1971). *Eleanor and Franklin: The story of their relationship based on Eleanor Roosevelt's private papers.* New York, NY: Norton.

Lash, J. P. (1972). *Eleanor: The years alone.* New York, NY: Norton.

Laudan, L. (1990). *Science and relativism: Some key controversies in the philosophy of science.* Chicago, IL: University of Chicago Press.

Licht, S. (1950). The principles of occupational therapy. In W. R. Dunton, & S. Licht (Eds.), *Occupational therapy principles and practice* (pp. 8–19). Springfield, IL: Thomas.

Licht, S. (1952). Writing the scientific paper. *American Journal of Occupational Therapy, VI,* 55–157.

Litterist, T. A. (1992). Occupational therapy: The role of ideology in the development of a profession for women. *American Journal of Occupational Therapy, 46,* 20–25.

Llorens, L. A. (1960). Psychological tests in planning therapy goals. *American Journal of Occupational Therapy, XIV,* 243–246.

Llorens, L. A. (1967a). An evaluation procedure for children 6 to 10 years of age. *American Journal of Occupational Therapy, XXI,* 64–69.

Llorens, L. A. (1967b). Projective techniques in occupational therapy. *American Journal of Occupational Therapy, XXI,* 226–229.

Llorens, L. A. (1968a). Changing methods in the treatment of psychosocial dysfunction. *American Journal of Occupational Therapy, XXII,* 26–29.

Llorens, L. A. (1968b). Identification of Ayres syndrome in children with behavior maladjustment. *American Journal of Occupational Therapy, XXII,* 286–288.

Llorens, L. A. (1970). Facilitating growth and development: The promise of occupational therapy. *American Journal of Occupational Therapy, XXIV,* 93–101.

Llorens, L. A. (1972). Problem-solving the role of occupational therapy in a new environment. *American Journal of Occupational Therapy, 26,* 234–238.

Llorens, L. A. (1973). Occupational therapy in the community. *American Journal of Occupational Therapy, 27*(8), 453–456.

Llorens, L. A. (1974a). The effects of stress on growth and development. *American Journal of Occupational Therapy, 28,* 82–86.

Llorens, L. A. (1974b). Learning disability, occupational therapy and community programming. Proceeding of the 6th International Congress: World Federation of Occupational Therapy, Vancouver, British Columbia, Canada, August 12–16, 1974, pp. 262–274.

Llorens, L. A. (1976). *Application of a developmental theory for health and rehabilitation.* Rockville, MD: American Occupational Therapy Association.

Llorens, L. A. (1977). A developmental theory revisited. *American Journal of Occupational Therapy, 31,* 656–657.

Llorens, L. A. (1981a). A journal in research in occupational therapy: The need, the response. *Occupational Therapy Journal of Research, 1,* 3–6.

Llorens, L. A. (1981b). Occupational therapy: State of the art-potential for development. Unpublished paper presented at the New Zealand Association of Occupational Therapists, August 26–29, 1981, Auckland, New Zealand.

Llorens, L. A. (1984). Changing balance: Environment and individual. *American Journal of Occupational Therapy, 38,* 30–34.

Llorens, L. A. (1990). Research utilization: A personal/professional responsibility. *Occupational Therapy Journal of Research, 10,* 3–6.

Llorens, L. A., & Bernstein, S. P. (1963). Finger painting with an obsessive-compulsive organically-damaged child. *American Journal of Occupational Therapy, XVII,* 120–121.

Llorens, L. A., & Gillette, N. P. (1985). The challenge for research in a practice profession. *American Journal of Occupational Therapy, 39*(3), 143–146.

Llorens, L. A., Levy, R., & Rubin, E. Z. (1964). Work adjustment program: A pre-vocational experience. *American Journal of Occupational Therapy, XVIII,* 15–19.

Llorens, L. A., & Rubin, E. Z. (1962). A directed activity program for disturbed children. *American Journal of Occupational Therapy, XVI,* 287–307.

Llorens, L. A., Rubin, E. Z., Braun, J., Beck, G., Mottley, N., & Beall, D. (1964). Cognitive-perceptual-motor functions: A preliminary report on training. *American Journal of Occupational Therapy, XVIII,* 202–208.

Llorens, L. A., & Snyder, N. V. (1987). Research initiative for occupational therapy. *American Journal of Occupational Therapy, 41,* 491–493.

Ludmerer, K. M. (1999). *Time to heal: American medical education.* New York, NY: Oxford University Press.

Ludwig, F. M. (1988a). Gail Fidler. In R. Miller, K. Sieg, F. Ludwig, S. D. Shortridge, & J. Van Deusen (Eds.), *Six perspectives on theory for the practice of occupational therapy* (pp. 17–39). Rockville, MD: Aspen.

Ludwig, F. M. (1988b). Anne Cronin Mosey. In R. Miller, K. Sieg, F. Ludwig, S. D. Shortridge, & J. Van Deusen (Eds.), *Six perspectives on theory for the practice of occupational therapy* (pp. 41–61). Rockville, MD: Aspen.

Manley, J. E. (1995). Sex-segregated work in the system of professions: The development and stratification of nursing. *The Sociological Quarterly, 32*(2), 297–314.

Marius, R. (1999). *A short guide to writing about history.* New York, NY: Longman.

Mathewson, M. (1975). Female and married: Damaging to the therapy profession? *American Journal of Occupational Therapy, 29,* 601–607.

May, E. T. (1988). *Homeward bound: American families in the Cold War.* New York, NY: Basic Books.

Mazer, J. L., Fidler, G. S., Kovalenko, L., & Overly, K. (1968). Exploring how a think feels. Selected portions of a workshop on object relations theory in occupational therapy held at waldenwoods conference center, May 26–31, 1968, Hartland, MI. Sponsored by the American Occupational Therapy Association under Grant No.

123-T-68 from the Rehabilitation Services Administration, Social and Rehabilitation Services, United States Department of Health, Education and Welfare.

McNary, H. (1954). The scope of occupational therapy. In H. S. Willard & C. S. Spackman (Eds.), *Principles of occupational therapy* (2nd ed., pp. 11–23). Philadelphia, PA: Lippincott.

Meyer, A. (1922). The philosophy of occupational therapy. *Archives of Occupational Therapy, 1,* 1–10.

Morantz-Sanchez, R. M. (1985). *Sympathy and science: Women physicians in American medicine.* New York, NY: Oxford University Press.

Morantz-Sanchez, R. M. (1997). Female science and medical reform: A path not taken. In R. G. Walters (Ed.), *Scientific authority and twentieth century America* (pp. 99–116). Baltimore, MD: Johns Hopkins University Press.

Mosey, A. C. (1968a). Occupational therapy: Theory and practice. Training program supported in part by training grant No. 543-T-65 from the Rehabilitation Services Administration, Department of Health, Education and Welfare, Washington, D. C. to the Medical Foundation, Inc. in collaboration with Massachusetts Department of Mental Health. Medford, MA: Pothier Brothers, Printers, Inc.

Mosey, A. C. (1968b). Recapitulation of ontogenesis: A theory of occupational therapy practice. *American Journal of Occupational Therapy, XXII,* 426–432.

Mosey, A. C. (1971). Involvement in the rehabilitation movement 1942–1960. *American Journal of Occupational Therapy, XXV,* 234–236.

Mosey, A. C. (1973). *Activities therapy.* New York, NY: Raven.

Mosey, A. C. (1981). *Occupational therapy: Configuration of a profession.* New York, NY: Raven.

Mosey, A. C. (1985). Eleanor Clarke Slagle lecture: A monistic or a pluralistic approach to professional identity? *American Journal of Occupational Therapy, 39,* 504–509.

Mosey, A. C. (1986). *Psychosocial components of occupational therapy.* New York, NY: Raven.

Mosey, A. C. (1993). Partition of occupational science and occupational therapy: Sorting out some issues. *American Journal of Occupational Therapy, 47,* 751–754.

Mosey, A. C. (1996). *Applied scientific inquiry in the health professions: An epistemological orientation.* Bethesda, MD: American Occupational Therapy Association.

Mosey, A. C. (1998). The competent scholar. *American Journal of Occupational Therapy, 52,* 760–764.

National Organization for Woman (1966). NOW statement of purpose. In R. Griffith (Ed.), *Major problems in American history since 1945* (pp. 507–509). Lexington, MA: D. C. Health Company.

Neuenschwander, J. A. (2002). *Oral history and the law: Practices in oral history.* Carlisle, PA: Oral history association, Dickinson College.

Oral History Association. (2001). *Oral history evaluation guidelines.* Adopted 1989, revised 2000. Carlisle, PA: Author.

Ottenbacher, K. J. (1987). Research: Its importance to clinical practice in occupational therapy. *American Journal of Occupational Therapy, 41,* 213–215.

Ottenbacher, K. J. (1992). Confusion in occupational therapy research: Does the end justify the method? *American Journal of Occupational Therapy, 46,* 871–874.

Oyster, C. K., Hanten, W. P., & Llorens, L. A. (1987). *Introduction to research: A guide for the health service professional*. Philadelphia, PA: Lippincott.

Parham, L. D. (1998). What is the proper domain of occupational therapy research? *American Journal of Occupational Therapy, 52*, 485–489.

Perkins, K. B. (1991). Book review. [Review of the book *The system of professions: An essay on division of expert labor*.]. *Sociological Inquiry, 61*(1), 124–126.

Peters, C. O. (1987). Graduate education in occupational therapy: Historical synthesis. Unpublished master's project report. San Jose State University, San Jose, CA.

Plato. (1976). *Meno*. (G. M. A. Grube Trans.). Indianapolis, IN: Hackett.

Polit, D. F., & Hungler, B. P. (1995). *Nursing research, principles and methods*. Philadelphia, PA: Lippincott.

Quiroga, V. (1995). *Occupational therapy: The first 30 years 1900 to 1930*. Bethesda, MD: American Occupational Therapy Association.

Rampolla, M. L. (2001). *A pocket guide to writing history*. Boston, MA: Bedford/St. Martin's Press.

Reed, K. L. (1986). Tools of practice: Heritage or baggage? *American Journal of Occupational Therapy, 40*, 597–605.

Reed, K. L., & Sanderson, S. N. (1999). *Concepts of occupational therapy*. Philadelphia, PA: Lippincott Williams & Wilkins.

Reilly, M. (1960). Research potentiality of occupational therapy. *American Journal of Occupational Therapy, XIV*, 206–209.

Reilly, M. (1962). Occupational therapy can be one of the great ideas of 20th century medicine. *American Journal of Occupational Therapy, XVI*, 1–9.

Reilly, M. (1966). A psychiatric occupational therapy program as a teaching model. *American Journal of Occupational Therapy, 20*, 61–67.

Reilly, M. (1969). The educational process. *American Journal of Occupational Therapy, 23*, 299–307.

Reilly, M. (1971). The modernization of occupational therapy. *American Journal of Occupational Therapy, XXV*, 243–246.

Reilly, M. (1974). *Play as exploratory learning: Studies of curiosity behavior*. Beverly Hills, CA: Sage.

Reverby, S. M. (1987). *Ordered to care: The dilemma of American nursing, 1850–1945*. New York, NY: Cambridge University Press.

Ritchie, D. A. (1995). *Doing oral history*. New York, NY: Twayne.

Ritchie, D. A. (2003). *Doing oral history: A practical guide*. New York, NY: Oxford University Press.

Robertson, S. C. (1988). *Mental health focus: Skills for assessment and treatment*. Rockville, MD: American Occupational Therapy Association.

Robertson, S. C. (1992). *Find a mentor or be one*. Rockville, MD: American Occupational Therapy Association.

Rogers, J. C. (1982). Order and disorder in medicine and occupational therapy. *American Journal of Occupational Therapy, 36*, 29–35.

Rogers, J. C. (1983). Clinical reasoning: The ethics, science and art. *American Journal of Occupational Therapy, 37*, 601–616.

Rosenow, A. M. (1982). Without a wife: The dilemma of social support for women's careers. In J. Muff, (Ed.), *Socialization, sexism and stereotyping: Women's issues in nursing* (pp. 281–289). St. Louis, MO: Mosby.

Rossiter, M. W. (1995). *Women scientists in America: Before affirmative action 1940–1972*. Baltimore, MD: Johns Hopkins University Press.

Rozier, C. (1994). Power and pt's. *PT Magazine*, Nov, 42–46.

Scardina, V. (1981). From pegboards to integration. *American Journal of Occupational Therapy, 35*, 581–588.

Schein, E. H. (1972). *Professional education: Some new directions*. New York, NY: McGraw–Hill.

Schemm, R. L., & Bross, T. (1995). Mentorship experiences in a group of occupational therapy leaders. *American Journal of Occupational Therapy, 49*, 32–37.

Schon, C. (1983). *The reflective practitioner: How professions think in action.* New York, NY: Basic Books.

Schwartz, K. B. (1992a). Examining profession's legacy. *American Journal of Occupational Therapy, 46*, 9–10.

Schwartz, K. B. (1992b). Occupational therapy and education: A shared vision. *American Journal of Occupational Therapy, 46*, 12–18.

Schwartz, K. B., & Colman, W. (1988). Historical research methods in occupational therapy. *American Journal of Occupational Therapy, 42*, 239–244.

Serrett, K. D. (1985). Another look at occupational therapy's history: Paradigm or pair-of-hands. In K. D. Serrett (Ed.), *Philosophical and historical roots of occupational therapy* (pp. 1–31). New York, NY: Haworth.

Shannon, P. (1977). The derailment of occupational therapy. *American Journal of Occupational Therapy, 31*, 229–234.

Shannon, P. D. (1983). Toward a philosophy of occupational therapy. Prepared from the Report on the Project to Identify the Philosophy of Occupational Therapy, January, 1983. Conducted under the auspices of the American Occupational Therapy Association, Rockville, MD. In private collection of R. K. Bing.

Shannon, P. (1993). Philosophical consideration for the practice of occupational therapy. In S. E. Ryan (Ed.), *The certified occupational therapy assistant* (pp. 35–42). Thorofare, NJ: Slack.

Simpson, R. L., & Simpson, I. H. (1969). Women and bureaucracy in the semi-professions. In A. Etzioni (Ed.), *The semi-professions and their organizations: Teachers, nurses and social workers* (pp. 196–265). New York, NY: Free Press.

Solomon, B. M. (1985). *In the company of educated women: A history of women and higher education in America*. New Haven, CT: Yale University Press.

Spackman, C. S. (1954). Occupational therapy for patients with physical disabilities: Part I. In H. S. Willard, & C. S. Spackman (Eds.), *Principles of Occupational Therapy*, (2nd ed., pp. 168–257). Philadelphia, PA: Lippincott.

Spradley, J. P. (1979). *The ethnographis interview*. Belmont, CA: Wadsworth.

Starr, D. (1982). *The social transformation of American medicine*. New York, NY: Basic Books.

Stattel, F. M. (1952). Occupational therapy department Kessler Institute. *American Journal of Occupational Therapy, VI*, 29–30.

Stattel, F. M. (1954). The painful phantom limb. *American Journal of Occupational Therapy, VIII*, 156–157.

Stattel, F. M. (1956). Equipment designed for occupational therapy. *American Journal of Occupational Therapy, X*, 194–204.

Stattel, F. M. (1966). The occupational therapist in rehabilitation: Projections toward the future. *American Journal of Occupational Therapy, XX,* 144–146.

Stattel, F. M. (1977). Sense of the past-focus on the present. *American Journal of Occupational Therapy, 31,* 649–650.

Steinem, G. (1994). *Moving beyond words.* New York, NY: Simon and Schuster.

Storey, W. K. (1999). *Writing history: A guide for students.* New York, NY: Oxford University Press.

Tapper, B. E. (1991). USC Pays highest tribute to Elizabeth Yerxa. *OT Week,* April 4, 1991, p. 2.

Tobias, S. (1997). *Faces of feminism: An activist's reflection on the women's movement.* Boulder, CO: Westview Press.

Tomes, N. (1998). *The gospel of germs: Men, women and the microbe in American life.* Cambridge, MA: Harvard University Press.

Tuchman, B. W. (1981). *Practicing history: Selected essays.* New York, NY: Alfred A. Knopf.

Tucker, A. (1939). *Miss Susie Slagle's.* New York, NY: Harper.

Turk, D. (2004). *Bound by a mighty vow: Sisterhood and women's fraternities 1870–1920.* New York, NY: New York University Press.

Turner, B. S. (1989). Book review. [Review of the book *The system of professions: An essay on division of expert labor*]. *Sociology, 23*(3), 472–473.

Van Deusen, J. (1988). Mary Reilly. In R. Miller, K. Sieg, F. Ludwig, S. D. Shortridge, & J. Van Deusen (Eds.), *Six perspectives on theory for the practice of occupational therapy* (pp. 143–158). Rockville, MD: Aspen.

Vansina, J. (1985). *Oral tradition as history.* Madison, WI: University of Wisconsin Press.

Veblen, T. (1994). *The theory of the leisure class.* New York, NY: Penguin. (Original work published 1899).

Viseltear, E. (1975). In this issue. *American Journal of Occupational Therapy, 29,* 641.

Walters, R. G. (1997). *Scientific authority and twentieth-century America.* Baltimore, MD: Johns Hopkins University Press.

Welles, C. (1952). Body mechanics of the bed patient as related to occupational therapy. *American Journal of Occupational Therapy, VI,* 197–202.

Welles, C. (1958). Da Vinci is dead: The case for specialization. *American Journal of Occupational Therapy, XII,* 289–290.

Welles, C. (1962). Administration: Do it yourself. *American Journal of Occupational Therapy, XVI,* 72–75.

Welles, C. (1969). The implications of liability: Guideline for professional practice. *American Journal of Occupational Therapy, XXIII,* 18–26.

Welles, C. (1976). Ethics in conflict: Yesterday's standards-outdated guide for tomorrow? *American Journal of Occupational Therapy, 30,* 44–47.

Welles, C. (1979). Specialization: Legal and administrative implications. *American Journal of Occupational Therapy, 33,* 118–119.

Welles, C. (1984). Liability considerations in the occupational therapy practice environment. In F. S. Cromwell (Ed.), *Occupational therapy strategies and adaptations for independent daily living* (pp. 35–45). New York, NY: Haworth.

Welles, C. (1985). Ethics and related professional liability. In J. Bair & M. Gray (Eds.), *The occupational therapy manager* (pp. 359–382). Rockville, MD: American Occupational Therapy Association.

West, W. (1959). Psychiatric Occupational Therapy. Proceedings of the Allenberry workshop conference on the function and preparation of the psychiatric occupational therapy, Allenberry Inn, November 13–19, 1956, Boiling Springs, PA. New York: American Occupational Therapy Association.

West, W. (1979). Historical perspectives. In Occupational therapy: 2001, papers presented at the special session of the representative assembly, November 8–12, 1978, in Scottsdale, AZ, (pp. 9–17). Rockville, MD: American Occupational Therapy Association.

West, W. (1981). Commentary: A journal of research in occupational therapy, the response, the responsibility. *Occupational Therapy Journal of Research, 1*, 7–12.

West, W. (1991). A tribute to Lela Llorens. *OT Week, 11*, 10–11.

West, W. (1992). Ten milestone issues in AOTA history. *American Journal of Occupational Therapy, 46*, 1066–1074.

Wiemer, R. B. (1972a). What is the national health council? Is AOTA's membership in it worthy of budget priority? *American Journal of Occupational Therapy, 26*, 3A–4A.

Wiemer, R. B. (1972b). Some concepts of prevention as an aspect of community health: A foundation for development of the occupational therapists's role. *American Journal of Occupational Therapy, 26*, 1–9.

Wiemer, R. B. (1978). Traditional and nontraditional practice arenas. In *Occupational Therapy 2001* (pp. 42–53). Rockville, MD: American Occupational Therapy Association.

Wiemer, R. B., & West, W. L. (1970). Occupational therapy in community health care. *American Journal of Occupational Therapy, XXIV*, 323–328.

Wiesen-Cook, B. (1992). *Eleanor Roosevelt: Volume one 1884–1933*. New York, NY: Viking.

Wilensky, H., & Lebeau, C. (1965). *Industrial society and social welfare: Russell Sage Foundation*. New York, NY: Macmillan.

Willard, H. S., & Spackman, C. S. (1947). *Principles of occupational therapy*. Philadelphia, PA: Lippincott.

Wolcott, H. F. (2001). *Writing up qualitative research*. Thousand Oaks, CA: Sage.

Yerxa, E. J. (1967a). Authentic occupational therapy. *American Journal of Occupational Therapy, XXI*, 1–9.

Yerxa, E. J. (1967b). The American occupational therapy foundation is born. *American Journal of Occupational Therapy, XXI*, 299–300.

Yerxa, E. J. (1974). Occupational therapy research in 1974: Models of enlightment. Proceedings of the 6th International Congress: World Federation of Occupational Therapists, Vancouver, British Columbia, Canada, August 12–16, 1974, pp. 674–681.

Yerxa, E. J. (1975). On being a member of a feminine profession. *American Journal of Occupational Therapy, 29*, 597–598.

Yerxa, E. J. (1978). The occupational therapist as consultant and researcher. In H. L. Hopkins & H. D. Smith (Eds.), *Willard and Spackman's occupational therapy*, (5th ed., pp. 689–693).

Yerxa, E. J. (1979). The philosophical base of occupational therapy. In Occupational therapy: 2001, Papers presented at the special session of the representative assembly, November 8–12, 1978, in Scottsdale, AZ, (pp. 26–30). Rockville, MD: American Occupational Therapy Association.

Yerxa, E. J. (1980). Occupational therapy's role in creating a future climate of caring. *American Journal of Occupational Therapy, 34*, 529–534.

Yerxa, E. J. (1981). Basic or applied? A developmental assessment of occupational therapy research in 1981. *American Journal of Occupational Therapy, 35*, 820–821.

Yerxa, E. J. (1982). A response to testing and measurement in occupational therapy: A review of current practice with special emphasis on the southern California sensory integration tests. *American Journal of Occupational Therapy, 36*, 399–404.

Yerxa, E. J. (1983a). Research priorities. *American Journal of Occupational Therapy, 37*, p. 699.

Yerxa, E. J. (1983b). Audacious values: The energy source for occupational therapy practice. In G. Kielhofner (Ed.), *Health through occupation theory and practice in occupational therapy* (pp. 149–162). Philadelphia, PA: F. A. Davis.

Yerxa, E. J. (1983c). The occupational therapist as a researcher. In H. L. Hopkins & H. D. Smith (Eds.) *Willard and Spackman's occupational therapy*, (6th ed., pp. 869–875).

Yerxa, E. J. (1986). Target tomorrow. In *Target occupational therapy education: Promoting excellence in education* (pp. 209–213). Rockville, MD: American Occupational Therapy Association.

Yerxa, E. J. (1987). Research: The key to the development of occupational therapy as an academic discipline. *American Journal of Occupational Therapy, 41*, 415–419.

Yerxa, E. J. (1991). Seeking a relevant, ethical and realistic way of knowing occupational therapy. *American Journal of Occupational Therapy, 45*, 199–204.

Yerxa, E. J. (1992). Some implications of occupational therapy's history for its epistemology, values and relationship to medicine. *American Journal of Occupational Therapy, 46*, 79–83.

Yerxa, E. J. (1995). Who is the keeper of occupational therapy's practice and knowledge. *American Journal of Occupational Therapy, 49*, 295–299.

Yerxa, E. J. (1998). Occupation: The keystone for a self-defined profession. *American Journal of Occupational Therapy, 52*, 365–372.

Acknowledgements

Perhaps it is because I am an occupational therapist, I understand the power that a network or community, similar to the one I have studied, holds. This glimpse back to look forward in occupational therapy would not have been possible without the support that I have experienced in my professional and private life. Identifying specific individuals does not exclude the many conversations I have engaged in with numerous therapists and historians about the work. However, I am thankful to certain people for their individual support.

I would like to thank those therapists who provided introductions, liaisons, motivation, and unlocked doors to hidden historical treasures; Charles Christiansen, Martha Kirkland, Suzanne Peloquin, and now deceased Deborah Labovitz. Former Wilma L. West librarian and archivist, Mary Binderman, also assisted in uncovering valuable source materials.

Additionally there is a select group of scholars who challenged me to see the work in richer and more meaningful ways. Anne Cronin Mosey, whose early contributions to this study and my education served as a catalyst to my thinking and pursuit of scholarship. Marie-Louise Blount and Mary Donohue acted as expert consultants and readers.

Two historians mentored me to think beyond an internal view of occupational therapy. Diana Turk and Jonathan Zimmerman have contributed individually and collectively. Dr. Turk opened my eyes to the complexities of women's history, enriching my understanding of women's culture and contributions. Dr. Zimmerman, through his passion for history gave me the courage to press forward, enter his world, and challenged me to answer the harder questions. I am thankful for Jim Hinojosa, as an occupational therapy scholar and leader, for his unswerving dedication, and his vision of my worth and work.

Two women in my family, now deceased listened attentively as my thinking evolved, my mother and mother-in-law respectively, Marguerite Chorbajian, and Jeanette Harness. Finally, I would like to acknowledge my husband, Donald Peters, who provided the stamina and belief that occupational therapy history was worth the family sacrifices to support a work of this magnitude.

Christine Olga Peters, PhD, OTR/L, FAOTA Consultant
Sound Beach, New York

Index